Insomnia

About the Authors

William K. Wohlgemuth, PhD, graduated from the University of Miami with a degree in clinical health psychology. Following his internship, he completed postdoctoral training in the behavioral sleep medicine clinic at Duke University Medical Center. During that time, he was involved with several clinical trials investigating the efficacy of CBT-I. Since 2005, Dr. Wohlgemuth has been the director of the behavioral sleep medicine clinic at the Bruce W. Carter VA Medical Center in Miami. He is actively involved in training psychology practicum students and interns. Dr. Wohlgemuth is certified in behavioral sleep medicine by the American Academy of Sleep Medicine.

Ana Imia Fins, PhD, received her doctorate in clinical health psychology from the University of Miami. She completed predoctoral and postdoctoral training in behavioral sleep medicine at the Durham, NC, Veterans Affairs Medical Center and at the Duke University Sleep Disorders Center. Currently, she is professor at the College of Psychology at Nova Southeastern University, where she also codirects an insomnia clinic. For over 18 years she has been training students in the application of CBT-I and other behavioral sleep medicine intervention strategies.

Advances in Psychotherapy – Evidence-Based Practice

The basic objective of this series is to provide therapists with practical, evidence-based treatment guidance for the most common disorders seen in clinical practice – and to do so in a reader-friendly manner. Each book in the series is both a compact "how-to" reference on a particular disorder for use by professional clinicians in their daily work and an ideal educational resource for students as well as for practice-oriented continuing education.

The most important feature of the books is that they are practical and easy to use: All are structured similarly and all provide a compact and easy-to-follow guide to all aspects that are relevant in real-life practice. Tables, boxed clinical "pearls," marginal notes, and summary boxes assist orientation, while checklists provide tools for use in daily practice.

Continuing Education Credits

Psychologists and other healthcare providers may earn five continuing education credits for reading the books in the *Advances in Psychotherapy* series and taking a multiple-choice exam. This continuing education program is a partnership of Hogrefe Publishing and the National Register of Health Service Psychologists. Details are available at https://us.hogrefe.com/cenatreg

The National Register of Health Service Psychologists is approved by the American Psychological Association to sponsor continuing education for psychologists. The National Register maintains responsibility for this program and its content.

Advances in Psychotherapy – Evidence-Based Practice, Volume 42

Insomnia

William K. Wohlgemuth
Sleep Disorders Center, Bruce W. Carter VA Medical Center,
Miami, FL

Ana Imia Fins
College of Psychology, Nova Southeastern University,
Fort Lauderdale, FL

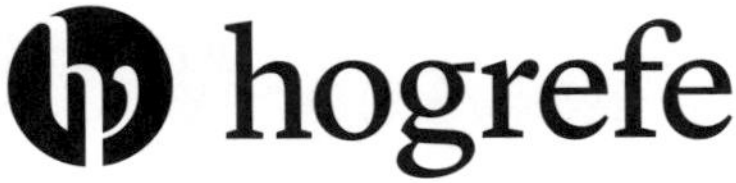

Library of Congress Cataloging in Publication information for the print version of this book is available via the Library of Congress Marc Database under the Library of Congress Control Number 2018960136

Library and Archives Canada Cataloguing in Publication
Wohlgemuth, William K., 1963-, author
Insomnia / William K. Wohlgemuth, Sleep Disorders Center, Bruce W. Carter VA Medical Center, Miami, FL, Ana Imia Fins, College of Psychology, Nova Southeastern University, Fort Lauderdale, FL. (Advances in psychotherapy--evidence-based practice ; v. 42)

Includes bibliographical references. Issued in print and electronic formats.
ISBN 978-0-88937-415-7 (softcover).--ISBN 978-1-61676-415-9 (PDF).--ISBN 978-1-61334-415-6 (EPUB)

1. Insomnia. 2. Insomnia--Treatment. 3. Insomniacs. I. Fins, Ana Imia, author II. Title. III. Series: Advances in psychotherapy--evidence-based practice ; v. 42

RC548.W64 2018 616.8'4982 C2018-906149-9
C2018-906150-2

http://www.hogrefe.com

PUBLISHING OFFICES

USA:	Hogrefe Publishing Corporation, 7 Bulfinch Place, Suite 202, Boston, MA 02114 Phone (866) 823-4726, Fax (617) 354-6875; E-mail customerservice@hogrefe.com
EUROPE:	Hogrefe Publishing GmbH, Merkelstr. 3, 37085 Göttingen, Germany Phone +49 551 99950-0, Fax +49 551 99950-111; E-mail publishing@hogrefe.com

SALES & DISTRIBUTION

USA:	Hogrefe Publishing, Customer Services Department, 30 Amberwood Parkway, Ashland, OH 44805 Phone (800) 228-3749, Fax (419) 281-6883; E-mail customerservice@hogrefe.com
UK:	Hogrefe Publishing, c/o Marston Book Services Ltd., 160 Eastern Ave., Milton Park, Abingdon, OX14 4SB, UK Phone +44 1235 465577, Fax +44 1235 465556; E-mail direct.orders@marston.co.uk
EUROPE:	Hogrefe Publishing, Merkelstr. 3, 37085 Göttingen, Germany Phone +49 551 99950-0, Fax +49 551 99950-111; E-mail publishing@hogrefe.com

OTHER OFFICES

CANADA:	Hogrefe Publishing, 660 Eglinton Ave. East, Suite 119-514, Toronto, Ontario, M4G 2K2
SWITZERLAND:	Hogrefe Publishing, Länggass-Strasse 76, 3012 Bern

Printed and bound in the USA

ISBN 978-0-88937-415-7 (print) • ISBN 978-1-61676-415-9 (PDF) • ISBN 978-1-61334-415-6 (EPUB)
http://doi.org/10.1027/00415-000

Preface

Insomnia is a widespread problem. Estimates suggest that, within a given year, about 40% of the population will experience difficulty falling or staying asleep, while about 10% experience chronic insomnia. Sleeping pills have been used for decades, but physicians are wary about the consequences of long-term use. Fortunately, efficacious nondrug, behavioral methods have been developed and tested over the past 2 decades. These treatments were developed with knowledge of the biological underpinnings of sleep. Additionally, during this time, investigators gained a better understanding of common beliefs about sleep and the disruptive habits which develop as a result of those beliefs. This knowledge has been incorporated into a treatment called *cognitive behavioral therapy for insomnia* (or CBT-I). Treatment guidelines based on reviews of the evidenced-based literature, published by both the American Academy of Sleep Medicine and the American College of Physicians, support CBT-I as first-line therapy for insomnia.

Insomnia is a common symptom of many medical, psychiatric, and other sleep disorders, and proper evaluation is necessary to rule out other potential causes of the sleep difficulty. Consultation with a sleep specialist may be needed to determine if a comorbid sleep disorder is present. Consultation with a physician or psychiatrist may be needed to rule out either medical or psychiatric causes of insomnia. Sometimes it may be necessary to work in tandem with a physician or sleep specialist to coordinate medical treatment (e.g., hypnotic medication) with CBT-I.

When learning any new therapeutic technique, therapists can be assisted by supervised practice for several cases to gain confidence in effective implementation of the therapy. We suggest that therapists seek to consult when beginning to use CBT-I, as clinical cases are varied and can be quite complex.

Our goal in this book is to provide a general overview of definitions, prevalence, impact, and theories of insomnia. We then provide a more specific, detailed description of the evaluation and treatment of insomnia. We also review more recent developments in the treatment of insomnia, such as the online implementation of CBT-I and interventions which focus more directly on cognitive aspects of insomnia. Recently, clinical trials have effectively combined CBT-I with other therapies (e.g., antidepressants) in patients with comorbid conditions (e.g., insomnia and depression). Positive results in these trials demonstrate the flexibility and strength of CBT-I with more complex presentations of insomnia.

Finally, we present a sample case of insomnia which includes the use of CBT-I. This case was not complicated with comorbidities and demonstrates many prototypical issues that arise when using CBT-I. The appendices include useful resources for assessment and treatment of insomnia, which readers are free to use in their practice.

Dedication

To my family – Mom and Dad, Kathy, Greg, and Mark – for their unconditional support and continued interest in my professional work.

W. K. W.

To my husband, Tony, who has always encouraged me to go outside my comfort zone and has steadfastly supported me in all of my professional endeavors; to Katrina and Anthony, whose love and support mean the world to me; and to my parents, who from an early age taught me to work hard and persevere in reaching my goals.

A. I. F.

Acknowledgments

We want to acknowledge our mentor and friend, Jack Edinger, PhD. Jack has been a pioneer and industrious investigator in behavioral sleep medicine. He introduced us to the world of insomnia during our internships and continued to train us in behavioral sleep medicine after hiring each of us as research coordinators for his insomnia grants. Since then, Jack has continued to mentor and serve as a consultant in our own work. We are both indebted to him for the fundamental role he has played in our professional development.

We are also grateful for the extensive encouragement and support received from Linda Sobell, PhD, even when our progress was impeded by unexpected events. Moreover, from the initial idea for this book and its inception, as well as throughout the writing process, her editorial feedback and comments have been invaluable and have greatly enhanced the clarity of the book.

Finally, we would like to acknowledge our students and their interest and excitement in learning how to diagnose and treat insomnia. Their energy has made it easy for us to "pay it forward" and emulate Jack's mentorship to train future behavioral sleep medicine specialists. We would also like to recognize Shantha Gowda and Danielle Millen for their contribution to the preparation of this book.

Contents

1

Description of Insomnia

1.1 Terminology

The term *insomnia* can be used to characterize a symptom, a cluster of symptoms, or a disorder. In broad terms, *insomnia* refers to difficulty sleeping. However, the complaints of insomnia can present in a variety of ways. Insomnia is characterized by difficulty either falling asleep or maintaining sleep (e.g., waking frequently during the night, difficulty falling asleep after waking, or awakening early in the morning without the ability to return to sleep). Sleep that is not restorative (in the absence of nighttime wakefulness) has historically been included as part of the diagnostic criteria. However, in the *Diagnostic and Statistical Manual of Mental Disorders* (5th ed.; DSM-5; American Psychiatric Association, 2013) the criteria for insomnia do not include nonrestorative sleep.

1.2 Definition

1.2.1 Classification of Insomnia

The characteristics of the symptoms can aid with the classification of the disorder and, in turn, can inform treatment planning. There are a number of different ways that symptoms of insomnia can be classified.

Insomnia associated with difficulty falling asleep, or initiating sleep, is classified as sleep-onset insomnia, whereas difficulty remaining asleep is considered sleep-maintenance insomnia. Most commonly, however, patients present with a combination of these sleep complaints.

Acute insomnia occurs at least 3 times per week and lasts less than 3 months

Insomnia can also be categorized by considering the duration of symptoms. *Acute insomnia* symptoms generally occur at least 3 times a week, last a brief period of time (less than 3 months; American Psychiatric Association, 2013), and are often easily linked to a precipitating cause (e.g., a significant life event). Symptoms associated with an acute episode often resolve without any type of intervention. Sometimes, however, the insomnia may be treated with a short trial of hypnotic medication to help the person manage troublesome symptoms. To be considered as chronic or persistent, insomnia complaints must be experienced at least three times per week for a minimum of 3 months. However, patients with *chronic insomnia* typically report symptoms that persist over a longer period of time.

Chronic insomnia lasts 3 months or more

Insomnia most often presents concurrently with medical or psychiatric conditions. In such cases, the insomnia disorder can be classified as a comorbid disorder. The term *primary insomnia* has been used to describe insomnia symptoms that cannot be attributed to another condition. However, the DSM-5 no longer utilizes the term *primary* to distinguish insomnia symptoms that are not linked to other conditions, from insomnia symptoms that occur concurrently with other disorders. When psychiatric, medical, or other sleep comorbidities exist, DSM-5 requires clinicians to specify and code the comorbid condition concurrently with the insomnia diagnosis (American Psychiatric Association, 2013). It is important to recognize that, in the case of comorbid insomnia, it is often difficult to ascertain the relationship between the insomnia symptoms and the concurrent disorder; as a result, establishing which condition presented first can be challenging. Differential diagnoses and comorbidities will be discussed further in Chapter 3 (Diagnosis, Assessment, and Treatment Indications).

When comorbidities exist, the diagnosis of insomnia can be more complicated

Three separate classification systems with diagnostic criteria for insomnia exist. These are the DSM-5, the *International Classification for Sleep Disorders* (3rd ed.; ICSD; American Academy of Sleep Medicine, 2014), and the *International Classification of Diseases* (11th ed., ICD-11; World Health Organization, 2018). Differences in the diagnostic criteria across these classification systems have varied over the years. Currently the DSM-5, ICSD-3, and ICD-11 share similar diagnostic criteria for insomnia.

Diagnostic criteria have consolidated many previous diagnoses into one of *insomnia disorder*

1.3 Epidemiology

1.3.1 Prevalence

The prevalence of insomnia can be evaluated by examining the rates of insomnia as a symptom or as a diagnosable disorder. The operational definitions used to define insomnia can lead to highly variable prevalence findings. In fact, prevalence rates can vary dramatically and have been reported to range anywhere between 4% and 50% (Wade, 2011). In an epidemiological survey of community-dwelling residents, approximately 42% of respondents reported at least one symptom of insomnia (sleep-onset, sleep-maintenance, early morning awakenings, or nonrestorative sleep; Walsh et al., 2011). When considering prevalence rates of insomnia as a disorder, rates can also vary as a result of the diagnostic criteria and classification system used, with rates between 3% and 22% reported (Ohayon & Reynolds, 2009; Roth et al., 2011).

Certain patient characteristics are also associated with greater prevalence of insomnia, including being female or older, as well as having comorbid medical or psychiatric conditions or being employed as a shift worker (Morin & Jarrin, 2013a, 2013b; Ohayon, 2002).

Insomnia disorder is more prevalent among women, older people, and those with comorbid conditions

1.3.2 Economic Impact of Insomnia

Insomnia can have a significant impact on costs associated with health care utilization, medication use, and other direct costs, as well as indirect costs, such as increased absenteeism and reduced work productivity. Wade (2011) estimated annual direct costs (e.g., medication use, health care utilization) associated with insomnia in the US to be US $14 billion, while indirect costs (e.g., missed work days) range between US $77 billion and $92 billion annually. Moreover, Kessler et al. (2011) reported that insomnia (after controlling for comorbid conditions) was associated with almost 8 days of lost work performance annually; these losses translate to about US $60 billion annually in lost productivity. Costs can also be incurred as a result of accidents and injuries related to insomnia. For example, in a study of 4,900 people, those with insomnia reported more accidents and errors in the workplace (Shahly et al., 2012). In addition, the authors found that costs associated with insomnia-related accidents and errors were significantly more costly than those not related to insomnia. Further, they estimated the cost of insomnia-related accidents and errors in employment settings to be approximately US $31 billion. Recently, Reynolds and Ebben (2017), using data adjusted for inflation, estimated combined direct and indirect costs of insomnia to range annually between US $150 billion and $175 billion, respectively.

Insomnia is associated with a costly loss of productivity and workplace accidents

When assessing the financial impact of insomnia, it is important to report the costs associated with treatment. Both *cognitive behavioral therapy for insomnia* (CBT-I) and *sedative-hypnotic treatments* have been shown to be cost-effective overall. However, head-to-head comparisons that account for combined direct and indirect cost-effectiveness, as well as costs associated with adverse effects, are difficult to find. Utilizing simulations to estimate costs for insomnia treatment in community-dwelling older adults, Tannenbaum et al. (2015) determined the cost to treat insomnia with sedative-hypnotic treatment would be US $32,452/person per year as compared with US $19,442 for CBT-I. These large estimated treatment costs included additional costs associated with the consequences of falls.

Reynolds and Ebben (2017) attempted to compare direct cost estimates for CBT-I and pharmacotherapy. Using 3 years as their calculation period (based on the longest period that CBT-I treatments have been examined), they calculated the cost of CBT-I to be slightly greater than that of pharmacotherapy (US $420 and $381, respectively.) They also noted that if medication use was continued for longer time periods (with corresponding physician visits for medication management), CBT-I would likely become more cost-effective than pharmacotherapy. These findings suggest that over the long term, when compared with pharmacotherapy, the use of CBT-I will be associated with reduced direct and indirect costs.

Use of CBT-I may be more cost-effective than medical management with sleeping pills

1.4 Course and Prognosis

The course of insomnia symptoms can be highly variable. For some patients, symptoms are short-lived while for others the course can be significantly protracted. Even in the case of chronic insomnia, the intensity of symptoms can vary significantly from night to night.

For many individuals, transient insomnia symptoms can remit without further exacerbation of symptomatology. However, numerous longitudinal studies show that a significant proportion of individuals with moderate to severe insomnia, as many as 80%, failed to show signs of remission over time (Mendelson, 1995; Morin, Bélanger et al., 2009; Morin & Jarrin, 2013a; Sateia, Doghramji, Hauri, & Morin, 2000).

Experts recommend immediate initiation of treatment once the diagnosis is established

Based on findings from a 3-year longitudinal study, Morin, Belanger et al. (2009) recommended initiating treatment immediately when patients present with sufficient symptoms to meet diagnostic criteria for insomnia, since improvement without treatment does not seem to occur. The American Academy of Sleep Medicine (AASM) has published clinical guidelines for the treatment of chronic insomnia (Schutte-Rodin, Broch, Buysse, Dorsey, & Sateia, 2008). These evidence-based guidelines provide recommendations for treatments that improve symptoms. In addition to the AASM, the American College of Physicians has reviewed the evidence from clinical trials and has recommended that CBT-I be utilized as the first line of treatment for chronic insomnia rather than sleeping pills (Qaseem, Kansagara, Forciea, Cooke, & Denberg, 2016). When properly evaluated, accurately diagnosed, and appropriately treated, insomnia has a prognosis that can be quite good.

Clinical Pearl
American College of Physicians Clinical Practice Guidelines

Recommendation 1: The American College of Physicians (ACP) recommends that all adult patients receive CBT-I as the initial treatment for chronic insomnia disorder.

Recommendation 2: ACP recommends that clinicians use a shared decision-making approach, including a discussion of the benefits, harms, and costs of short-term use of medications, to decide whether to add pharmacological therapy in adults with chronic insomnia disorder in whom CBT-I alone was unsuccessful (Qaseem, Kansagara, Forciea, Cooke, & Denberg, 2016, p. 125).

1.5 Differential Diagnosis of Insomnia From Other Sleep Disorders

Several sleep disorders may be accompanied by insomnia and should be assessed. These sleep disorders include restless legs syndrome, circadian rhythm sleep disorders (i.e., delayed or advanced sleep phase, shift work sleep disorder), sleep apnea, narcolepsy, sleepwalking, sleep eating, and substance- or medication-induced sleep disorder. Although each sleep disorder may present with insomnia as a complaint, all have specific diagnostic criteria to distinguish them from an insomnia disorder and may require further assessment and treatment by a sleep specialist. Differential diagnosis is important to accurately match interventions to the underlying causes of a sleep disorder.

Differential diagnosis of sleep disorders is important for proper intervention

Symptoms of *restless legs syndrome* include an urge to move one's legs, combined with uncomfortable leg sensations (Allen et al., 2003; Hening et al., 2004). These sensations follow a circadian pattern and typically peak at bedtime. Because of this pattern, restless legs more often interfere with sleep onset and should be considered in those with difficulty falling asleep (Allen et al., 2014).

Circadian rhythm disorders may present clinically as sleep-onset insomnia (delayed sleep phase) or early morning awakening (advanced sleep phase). Delayed and advanced sleep phase can be distinguished from insomnia disorder by observing that normal quantities of consolidated sleep are obtained, but the sleep period occurs either earlier (advanced) or later (delayed) than desired (Barion & Zee, 2007; Wyatt, 2004).

Fifty percent of sleep apnea patients complain of insomnia

Obstructive sleep apnea (OSA) is a breathing-related sleep disorder where the upper airway collapses repeatedly when sleeping (Epstein et al., 2009). These events cause brief obstructions to normal breathing and reduce oxygen levels in the body. Breathing is subsequently resumed through cortical arousal. In severe sleep apnea, this cycle may occur every 1–2 min during sleep. Most of the arousals that wake up these patients are not remembered, because the arousal may only last a few seconds. However, it is estimated that 50% of sleep apnea patients also complain of insomnia (Luyster, Buysse, & Strollo, 2010). These individuals experience longer bouts of wakefulness during their sleep period. *Polysomnography* (PSG; sometimes called a *sleep study*) is the physiological assessment required for the diagnosis of sleep apnea and should be considered if patients report loud snoring, are obese, and have been observed stopping breathing during their sleep.

Narcolepsy is a relatively rare sleep disorder that typically presents with extreme sleepiness during the wake period (Morgenthaler, Kapur, et al., 2007). These individuals persistently either fall asleep or struggle to stay awake during the day. In addition, these individuals may experience hallucinations at the beginning or end of their sleep period, and may also feel like they are unable to move upon awakening (sleep paralysis). Finally, muscle weakness (e.g., knees buckling, head drooping) in the context of a strong emotion is called *cataplexy* and may occur in patients with narcolepsy. Fragmented sleep occurs in most patients with narcolepsy, and they may have a few hours of waketime each night. If narcolepsy symptoms are present, these patients should be referred to a sleep center.

Parasomnias such as nightmares, sleepwalking, or sleep eating may cause awakenings and then create difficulty returning to sleep (Mahowald, Bornemann, & Schenck, 2004; Ohayon, Mahowald, Dauvilliers, Krystal, & Leger, 2012). Usually bedpartners or others sharing the home may be aware of these unusual nocturnal behaviors. If sleepwalking, sleep eating, night terrors, or other parasomnias appear to be the precipitant of the difficulty staying asleep, referral for further sleep evaluation should occur. Nightmares, in particular, with fear and anxiety related to terrifying dream content, can lead to wakefulness. Repeated unpleasant nightmare experiences may result in a conditioned arousal response that may exacerbate and perpetuate the sleep difficulty. In an epidemiological study of over 1,000 individuals with insomnia, nightmares were reported in 18% of the sample (Ohayon, Morselli, & Guilleminault, 1997). In a large community-based study, nightmares were significantly correlated with the presence of insomnia symptoms (Li, Zhang, Li, & Wing, 2010). Nightmare complaints presenting with insomnia should be evaluated, as they may interfere with the treatment of insomnia or may be a symptom of other psychiatric comorbidity such as posttraumatic stress disorder (PTSD).

Illicit substance use, alcohol consumption, or prescription medication use should always be considered during an insomnia assessment (Brower, 2003;

Morgan, Dixon, Mathers, Thompson, & Tomeny, 2003). Obviously, any substance with stimulant properties will interfere with sleep if used close to bedtime. Alcohol exerts paradoxical properties on sleep: It can facilitate sleep early in the sleep period, but later interfere with sleep (Roehrs & Roth, 2001). Prescribed medications also may interfere with sleep. For example, albuterol is a stimulant used to treat asthma which may cause insomnia. Stimulants used to treat attention-deficit disorder may also interfere with sleep. Caffeine usage should be assessed to determine its contribution to poor sleep.

Sleeping for short periods each night does not necessarily require a diagnosis of insomnia

A final consideration for differential diagnosis is normal variation in sleep patterns. Personal sleep needs vary, and some individuals are *short sleepers*. While these short sleepers may believe or have been told that they need more sleep, they do not experience daytime symptoms (e.g., no sleepiness or fatigue) after a short bout of sleep. Yet due to their belief that they require more sleep, they may spend more time in bed than necessary trying to get additional sleep. The additional time in bed will be spent awake and will be perceived by patients to be insomnia. Usually education about variation in sleep needs and reducing time in bed are helpful for such individuals. Please see the resource websites listed in Appendix 1.

1.6 Comorbidities

Consideration of other comorbidities is important to ensure appropriate treatment for each

Insomnia often presents concurrently with other conditions including medical conditions, psychiatric or substance use disorders, or other sleep disorders. While insomnia symptoms may overlap with the comorbid diagnosis (e.g., insomnia and depression) or appear to be a result of the comorbid diagnosis (e.g., insomnia in patients with chronic pain), recognizing insomnia as a separate comorbid disorder ensures appropriate treatment of both conditions.

1.6.1 Sleep Disorders Comorbidities

Although the previously described sleep disorders may be the primary cause of insomnia symptoms, more commonly insomnia exists as a separate (comorbid) sleep disorder that requires independent treatment. Referring individuals to a sleep center for evaluation and treatment of other sleep disorders may not necessarily improve their symptoms if the insomnia is not addressed.

OSA provides a good example of a sleep disorder that is often comorbid with insomnia. OSA is a breathing-related sleep disorder where the upper airway repeatedly collapses during sleep. These obstructions in the airway cause the sleeper to wake up so they will start breathing normally again. Fragmented sleep is the result of this recurring cycle of airway collapse and awakening throughout the night. Individuals with OSA usually are not aware that they have this problem, because they are asleep when the events occur. However, observation of loud snoring or breathing pauses from a bedpartner or excessive daytime sleepiness reported from the patient may indicate the presence of OSA. Diagnosis of OSA requires an overnight sleep study, and treatment of OSA requires specialized equipment (e.g., continuous positive airway pressure, or CPAP, machines), and these specialty diagnostic and treatment techniques require referral to a sleep center. The primary treatment for OSA is positive airway pressure, or PAP. This treatment introduces extra pressure in the upper airway so that it doesn't collapse during sleep. The most frequently used device is called continuous positive airway pressure or CPAP, which uses a single pressure while the patient is sleeping. Another device called BiPAP delivers two separate pressures, one for inhalation and another for exhalation. A third device is called AutoPAP continuously adjusts the pressure depending on the needs of the patient. In subsequent sections we will refer to the treatment for OSA as CPAP, but patients may be using one of the other devices.

Importantly, older adults with insomnia have OSA at a rate greater than the general population. Furthermore, nearly 50% of those who present with signs and symptoms of OSA have insomnia. Due to these high rates of comorbid insomnia and OSA, sleep difficulty should be reassessed after diagnosis of OSA has been made and treatment has been initiated. This reassessment is important because untreated insomnia frequently interferes with treatment adherence due to the fact that using a CPAP machine may be uncomfortable and lead to more wakefulness during the night (Ong & Crawford, 2013). From the CPAP user's perspective, the easiest solution to this problem is to not use CPAP. In this example of comorbid insomnia and OSA, leaving the insomnia untreated may lead to poor outcome for both conditions (untreated insomnia and OSA). However, treating the insomnia could improve consolidation of sleep and enhance adherence to CPAP therapy.

1.6.2 Medical Comorbidities

Rates of insomnia in those with medical conditions have been estimated to be as high as 86% (Glidewell, Moorcroft, & Lee-Chiong, 2010). Medical conditions that frequently present with comorbid insomnia symptoms include cancer, cardiovascular conditions (e.g., heart disease and hypertension), chronic obstructive pulmonary disease, arthritis, diabetes, ulcers, and neurological and menstrual problems (Budhiraja, Roth, Hudgel, Budhiraja, & Drake, 2011; Savard & Savard, 2013). In an epidemiological study of more than 1,700 individuals with medical conditions, Taylor et al. (2007) found that individuals with breathing problems, gastrointestinal problems, chronic pain, high blood pressure, and/or urinary problems were more likely to experience insomnia (even after adjusting for other sleep disorders, depression, and anxiety). Moreover, insomnia rates increased with increasing numbers of co-occurring medical conditions.

1.6.3 Psychiatric Comorbidities

Insomnia is the most common residual symptom following recovery from depression

Psychiatric conditions often present with comorbid insomnia complaints. Comorbidity rates for insomnia and psychiatric conditions have been estimated to range between 27% and 45% (Glidewell et al., 2010). One of the most common psychiatric diagnoses related to insomnia is depression, especially given that difficulty sleeping is a diagnostic criterion for *major depressive disorder*

(MDD). In a community sample, people with insomnia were almost 10 times more likely to have significant symptoms of depression (Taylor, Lichstein, Durrence, Reidel, & Bush, 2005). Further evidence for the comorbid nature of the two syndromes (rather than insomnia being merely a symptom of depression) comes from Carney, Segal, Edinger, and Krystal (2007), who found that after at least 20 weeks of either pharmacotherapy or cognitive behavioral therapy (CBT) for depression, approximately 50% of participants continued to report insomnia symptoms even when their depressive symptoms had remitted. Similarly, in a study examining residual symptoms after remission from MDD treated with pharmacotherapy, a large proportion of the sample (up to 58%) continued to experience some type of insomnia complaint after no longer meeting criteria for MDD (Nierenberg et al., 2010).

Generalized anxiety disorder (GAD) and panic disorder are often associated with sleep-onset and/or sleep-maintenance insomnia symptoms. In a large epidemiological study evaluating the comorbidity of insomnia with mental disorders, Ohayon, Caulet, and Lemoine (1998) found that comorbid sleep disturbance was greatest in individuals with GAD as compared with any other anxiety disorder evaluated. PSG studies also support sleep disruption in GAD and show that individuals with GAD (vs. controls) exhibit longer sleep-onset latencies, increased waketimes during sleep, decreased total sleep times, and reduced sleep efficiencies (Papadimitriou & Linkowski, 2005; Saletu-Zyhlarz et al., 1997). Similarly, among individuals with panic disorder, sleep panic attacks can contribute to sleep disruption, and anticipation of panic symptoms during sleep can produce sleep-onset and sleep-maintenance insomnia complaints (Mellman, 2006).

In addition to the comorbid relationships among depression, anxiety and insomnia, patients with more severe psychiatric conditions (e.g., PTSD, bipolar disorder, schizophrenia, or other psychotic disorders) often report insomnia symptoms (Soehner, Kaplan, & Harvey, 2013).

While insomnia can be present simultaneously with psychiatric disorders, some studies provide evidence that insomnia can predate psychiatric conditions and predict the development of a psychiatric disorder (Baglioni et al., 2011; Breslau, Roth, Rosenthal, & Andreski, 1996; Chang, Ford, Mead, Cooper-Patrick, & Klag, 1997; Ford & Kamerow, 1989).

1.7 Diagnostic Procedures

A comprehensive assessment is necessary to understand the nature of the insomnia for each patient

The diagnosis of insomnia requires a comprehensive evaluation that includes information regarding the nature of the problem (e.g., symptoms, symptom severity, history, and chronicity of symptoms), the consequences experienced (e.g., daytime fatigue, sleepiness), and the factors that may contribute to the symptoms (e.g., bedtime conditioned arousal, extended bedtimes; see Appendix 2) (Sateia et al., 2000). Additionally, an assessment of potential comorbid and differential conditions and diagnoses (e.g., mood disorders, other sleep disorders) is necessary. The preceding information is generally obtained through a thorough clinical interview and completion of self-report questionnaires. Detailed descriptions including the strengths and limitations of these assessment measures are addressed in Chapter 3 (Diagnosis, Assessment, and Treatment Indications).

A more detailed analysis of the sleep period is routinely obtained via a 2-week sleep diary (see Appendix 3). This allows for a real-time assessment of the patient's perception of the sleep complaint. In addition, sleep diaries can assist in ruling out other potential sleep conditions (e.g., circadian rhythm sleep disorders). It should be noted that actigraphs (small devices worn on the wrist that provide an objective assessment of movement and, in turn, an estimate of sleep and wake periods) and PSG are not routinely utilized in the assessment of insomnia (see Section 3.3: Other Methods of Assessing Sleep: Polysomnography and Actigraphy), although PSG can be indicated if differential diagnoses are required (Sateia et al., 2000).

2

Theories and Models of Insomnia

Multiple theoretical models exist to explain how insomnia develops and is maintained

Insomnia's development and maintenance has been conceptualized in various theoretical models. These models can assist in providing a rationale for a specific treatment formulation. This chapter will briefly describe early behavioral models of insomnia and then present newer models that have refined the earlier theories by incorporating cognitive perspectives. Early biological perspectives explaining insomnia that focus on physiological hyperarousal will also be described. These initial models serve as the foundation for a discussion of more recent neurobiological models of insomnia that are being proposed as advances in neuroimaging technology permit us to better understand brain function. Finally, a framework that integrates these multiple approaches to understanding insomnia will be presented. Before discussing the insomnia models, a brief description of the normal sleep–wake process will be presented.

2.1 Fundamentals of Sleep–Wake Regulation

Behavioral interventions often incorporate a psychoeducational module that provides a rationale for treatment to facilitate patients' acceptance of, and adherence to, treatment. Similarly, CBT-I integrates a psychoeducational component that incorporates concepts associated with the sleep process. The most widely used model of sleep–wake regulation, called the *two-process model*, is presented here to facilitate a basic understanding of the sleep process and factors that can impede normal sleep.

Borbély (1982) originally described a model that considers the effect of homeostatic processes and circadian influences on sleep and wakefulness. While the two separate processes independently contribute to sleepiness and wakefulness, they occur simultaneously and interact to produce regularity in the sleep–wake cycle.

2.1.1 Homeostatic Process

Sleep drive is an important biological regulator of the sleep process

The homeostatic process (called *Process S* by Borbely) is a mechanism by which a "sleep drive" or a propensity to fall asleep gradually develops. The longer an individual is awake, the greater is the drive to fall asleep. In turn, once a sleep period is initiated, the sleep drive gradually dissipates. In this context, an increase in the drive to sleep occurs as we spend more time awake.

This homeostatic process is driven by sleep-regulating substances, of which adenosine is the most widely studied. Adenosine is a by-product produced as energy is utilized by an active, waking brain. The longer an individual is awake, the more pronounced is the buildup of adenosine and other sleep-regulating substances. Eventually the drive to sleep is overwhelming, and under normal circumstances and without any external influences that might hinder this process, an individual falls asleep.

2.1.2 Circadian Process

The second process described by Borbely is the circadian process (referred to as *Process C*) that maintains the sleep–wake cycle occurring regularly in an overall period that lasts approximately 24 hrs. This process is driven by an internal clock residing in the suprachiasmatic nucleus of the hypothalamus. This internal clock drives many biological functions that oscillate in 24-hr cycles – for example, internal body temperature, level of arousal, and the release of cortisol. Daily synchronization or *entrainment* of this internal clock helps to ensure that this 24-hr regularity is maintained. This entrainment process occurs via exposure to sunlight and other cues that can provide synchronization (such as alarm clocks or meal times). Under normal circumstances, the circadian process influences sleep by synchronizing the sleep period to occur at approximately the same time every day.

An internal clock regulates many biological functions including sleep

2.1.3 Interaction of Homeostatic and Circadian Processes

Homeostatic and circadian processes interact with each other to either maintain wakefulness or induce sleep (Figure 1). As the homeostatic drive builds up throughout the day, the propensity to sleep increases. However, arousal level – driven by circadian influence – is also building up during the day, counterbalancing the sleep drive and helping to maintain wakefulness. Into the evening hours, the alertness provided by circadian factors begins to wane, and concomitantly with the increasing sleepiness fostered by the homeostatic sleep drive, sleep eventually is induced. Over the nighttime period as sleep progresses, the sleep drive associated with homeostatic factors diminishes and the rhythmicity of the circadian process begins to build up once more to facilitate wakefulness.

Sleep drive and circadian factors work together to regulate our alertness and sleepiness

While these two biological processes work automatically to maintain a regular sleep–wake cycle, many behaviors or activities can disrupt each process. For example, in the case of homeostatic sleep drive, consumption of caffeine can inhibit the effects of adenosine on the sleep system, and napping late in the day can reduce the buildup of sleep drive. Both of these actions can, in turn, delay the onset of sleep. In turn, the circadian process can be affected by significant daily schedule changes that routinely alter bedtimes and waketimes and, in turn, negatively affect the ability to get sleepy at the same time every night. Dysregulation of these underlying sleep–wake processes may interfere with the ability to fall asleep and stay asleep, and ultimately precipitate insomnia.

Dysregulation of sleep drive and circadian factors can interfere with a normal sleep rhythm

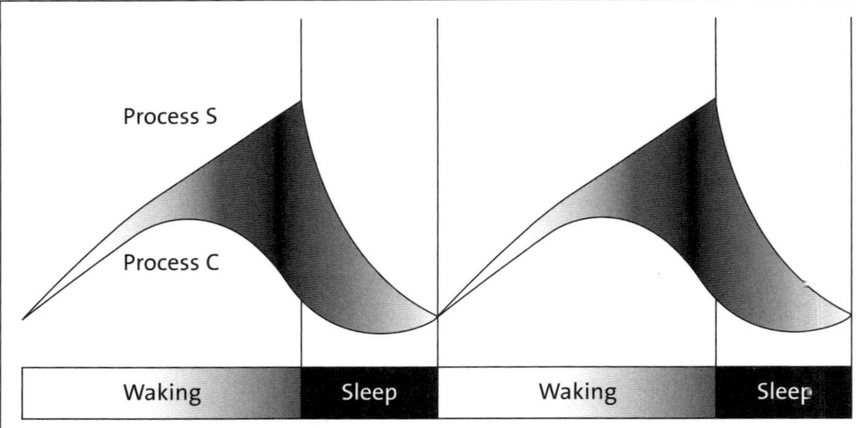

Figure 1
The two-process model for regulation of the sleep–wake cycle. Process S represents the need for sleep, which increases during wake and decreases during sleep. Process C represents the circadian system, which oscillates with a period of about 24 hrs. In this view, the times of sleep and wakefulness occur at the peak and trough of these additive processes, respectively. Reprinted with permission from "Circadian and Homeostatic Factors in Arousal" by R. Silver and J. LeSauter, 2008, *Annals of the New York Academy of Sciences, 1129*, p. 258. © 2008 by Wiley-Blackwell

2.2 Behavioral Model of Insomnia

High arousal combined with incompatible sleep behaviors can become cues for wakefulness in bed

The popularity of behaviorism in the 1960s and 1970s influenced thinking about the development of insomnia symptoms. Bootzin (1972) proposed a model of insomnia based on principles of learning theory, and more specifically, operant conditioning. His conceptualization proposed that falling asleep is an instrumental act designed to yield reinforcement – that is, sleep. Any stimulus associated with sleep (e.g., bedroom, bed), therefore, can become a discriminative stimulus for sleep. Bootzin proposed that in insomnia, the stimulus control for sleep is lacking, or alternatively, there are discriminative stimuli present that are not compatible with sleep behavior. In essence, the environment and stimuli that are traditionally associated with sleep are no longer discriminative stimuli for sleep behaviors and instead are associated with wakefulness. For individuals experiencing insomnia, being awake in bed increases arousal and frustration which, in turn, leads to greater concern and anxiety about falling asleep and/or staying asleep. Moreover, behaviors such as tossing and turning in bed, watching the clock constantly, and catastrophizing about lack of sleep occur frequently. During this process, the surrounding environment begins to be associated with the unpleasant experience of being awake, and stimuli that normally should be discriminative for sleep (such as the bed or bedroom) are no longer soporific and become discriminative cues for wakefulness. Often individuals with insomnia will report feeling sleepy in the moments leading up to bedtime only to find themselves wide awake once in bed. Their sleep environment becomes associated with cues associated with wakefulness. This is often referred to as *conditioned arousal*. It is not uncommon for these individuals to report much better sleep when they find themselves sleeping outside of their habitual sleep environment (e.g., a different room, in a hotel), as these other settings do not contain the conditioned stimuli for wakefulness that exist in their normal sleeping environment. This model is widely accepted by sleep specialists, and CBT-I generally incorporates stimulus control techniques to extinguish the arousal experienced in the normal sleep environment.

2.3 Cognitive Models of Insomnia

Various cognitive models have been proposed to explain underlying cognitive processes that may predispose an individual to insomnia or perpetuate its symptoms. In parallel with psychology's recognition of the importance of the role cognitions play in influencing behavior, Morin (1993) described the role of sleep-related dysfunctional beliefs and attitudes in perpetuating insomnia symptoms. For example, he reported that intrusive thoughts, worry, and negatively valenced cognitions are often present in insomnia. Specifically, his model identifies various cognitive constructs that contribute to cognitive, emotional, and physiological arousal and, in turn, promote maladaptive habits and sleep-incompatible behaviors. Cognitive errors (e.g., catastrophizing, magnification), unrealistic expectations associated with sleep, and misattributions about daytime impairment related exclusively to the effects of sleep loss are all considered significant contributors to anxiety and counterproductive behaviors that perpetuate sleep disruption. An individual with insomnia may, for example, believe that if they are unable to obtain 8 hrs of sleep, they must stay in bed longer the next morning to catch up on sleep, or take a nap during the day. These compensatory behaviors can lead to further disruption of sleep and greater psychological distress due to the discrepancy faced between the expectations and dysfunctional beliefs about sleep that are held by the individual and the disruption of sleep being experienced. Morin's model was one of the first to combine cognitive and behavioral approaches to the treatment of insomnia.

Harvey (2002, 2005) has further refined the role and emphasized the importance of cognitions by proposing a model that accounts for both nighttime and daytime cognitive processes in perpetuating insomnia symptoms. Nighttime factors include excessive negatively valenced cognitive activity, physiological arousal in conjunction with emotional distress, selective attention of sleep-related cues, unhelpful beliefs regarding sleep, distorted perception about sleep, and safety behaviors to avoid sleep loss.

Unlike other models that have focused primarily on nighttime factors, Harvey's model hypothesizes that the same processes operating at night also occur during the day. For example, selectively attending at night to bodily sensations that signal sleep onset may disrupt sleep, while in the daytime, selectively attending to signs that could be interpreted as resulting from poor sleep will increase worry about the potential consequences of poor sleep. Harvey's model serves as the foundation for a cognitive approach to the treatment of insomnia. Unlike the Morin model, in which both dysfunctional beliefs and maladaptive behaviors are addressed, the primary target of Harvey's model is altering cognitions.

Cognitive models emphasize maladaptive beliefs, safety behaviors, and increased arousal

More recently, models that emphasize metacognitive processes have been proposed to further refine cognitive models of insomnia. Ong, Ulmer, and Manber (2012) present a model that focuses on a two-level model of cognitive arousal. In this model, the first level of arousal, *primary arousal*, emphasizes cognitive processes that directly relate to sleep loss (e.g., dysfunctional beliefs about sleep needs or the impact of sleep loss). *Secondary arousal* refers to the awareness one has regarding sleep-related cognitions and serves to prime or bias the attention to sleep-related cognitions that occur at the primary level of arousal.

Several dimensions of secondary arousal are proposed by Ong et al. These include bias, rigidity, attachment, and absorption, and each is associated with primary arousal sleep-related cognitions. Ong and colleagues suggest that by focusing on biased processing of sleep-related thoughts and maintaining an inflexible perspective regarding sleep loss, primary and secondary arousal processes serve to precipitate and perpetuate insomnia symptoms. Metacognitive models are associated with *third-wave* therapies (e.g., mindfulness, acceptance, and commitment) that are now being explored in the context of insomnia treatment (Taylor, Hailes, & Ong, 2015).

2.4 Physiological Hyperarousal Models

Cognitive models posit that cognitive and/or emotional arousal is an important factor in insomnia. Other models emphasize excessive arousal in the central and peripheral nervous systems as a central feature of insomnia. Monroe (1967) was one of the earliest investigators to show that, compared with good sleepers, poor sleepers exhibited autonomic nervous system differences evidenced by significant elevations in rectal temperature, vasoconstriction, and skin resistance.

Physiological hyperarousal is considered to be a cause of insomnia

Other early studies have described elevations in muscle tension and core body temperature, suggesting that physiological arousal is a possible causal factor in the development of insomnia (Freedman & Sattler, 1982; Morris, Lack, & Dawson, 1990). The last 4 decades have witnessed considerable evidence supporting a physiological hyperarousal model of insomnia. Insomnia has been associated with alterations in cardiac indicators, stress-related hormones, and electroencephalogram (EEG) measures that reflect overactive central and peripheral nervous systems (for reviews, see Bonnet & Arand, 2010; Riemann et al., 2010).

2.5 A Neurocognitive Model

Perlis, Giles, Mendelson, Bootzin, and Wyatt (1997) integrated findings that support cortical (e.g., brain activity) hyperarousal to understand insomnia.

These authors conceptualized chronic insomnia as a result of cortical conditioned arousal in which high-frequency EEG activity (associated with activity in the gamma and beta ranges) is elevated in insomnia patients, particularly around the time of sleep onset. This excess cortical activation is associated with sensory experiences and cognitive processing that generally is reduced in good sleepers and may explain the difficulties experienced by insomniacs when attempting to fall asleep (as they are more vulnerable to arousal by external stimuli surrounding them). Moreover, this increased EEG activation may impede an individual's ability to discriminate between being awake and being asleep – perhaps via enhanced memory function. Indeed, it is not unusual for patients with insomnia to misperceive sleep as wakefulness during PSG sleep studies (Krystal, Edinger, Wohlgemuth, & Marsh, 2002). Perlis et al. (2001) propose that the higher-frequency beta EEG activity enhances memory around the time of sleep onset, despite the fact that normally this period would be susceptible to reduced memory recall. Enhanced memory around the periods of wake–sleep transitions may explain the frequent complaints of long sleep-onset latency (SOL) and long periods of wakefulness during the night reported by insomnia patients.

2.6 Neurobiological Models

Neuroscience is using new technology to provide evidence for the role that neural systems, composed of numerous brain structures, as well as localized groups of neural cells, play in insomnia. For example, Buysse, Germain, Hall, Monk, and Nofzinger (2012) proposed a neurobiological model to understand insomnia that incorporates regional brain circuits known to regulate sleep–wake processes. These brain circuits along with individual neurons and localized groups of neurons appear to be involved in the transition from wakefulness to sleep. Localized neurons release substances, such as adenosine, that regulate the activity of local and regional neurons and, in turn, control neural sleep–wake centers. Buysse et al. (2012) present data that confirm excessive activity during sleep in neural circuits and brain regions that are generally associated with wakefulness among insomnia patients as well as in animal models of insomnia. They propose that excessive activity in these areas may explain the subjective waking experiences reported by insomnia patients when PSG studies indicate sleep. Additionally, Buysse et al. note that lack of coordination among local sleep neurons may be related to limited or "partial" sleep states and may be responsible for diminished sleep quality in insomnia.

2.7 An Integrative Framework

Edinger and Means (2005; see Figure 2) developed a useful heuristic that integrates the previously described models of insomnia.

This model proposes that the clinical presentation of chronic insomnia derives from a combination of (a) dysfunctional cognitions, (b) homeostatic sleep drive dysregulation, (c) circadian disruption, and (d) other sleep inhibitory factors (e.g., conditioned arousal). The proposed model holds that dysfunctional beliefs and attitudes about sleep lead to new bedtime behaviors that, from a poor sleeper's perspective, are expected to improve daytime symptoms following poor sleep. These new bedtime behaviors may include spending 10 hrs in bed to get 8 hrs of sleep, or having a variable wake-up time that depends on the quality of the prior night's sleep. Although a poor sleeper may believe that these new behaviors will improve daytime dysfunction, these strategies are more likely to perpetuate poor sleep. This model makes explicit the complicated, multifactorial nature of the chronic insomnia problem. The heuristic in Figure 2 shows the relevance of both cognitive and behavioral factors and their disruption of homeostatic and circadian processes. Furthermore, these new behaviors may exacerbate other sleep inhibitory factors such as conditioned arousal.

Insomnia is a complicated, multifactorial problem

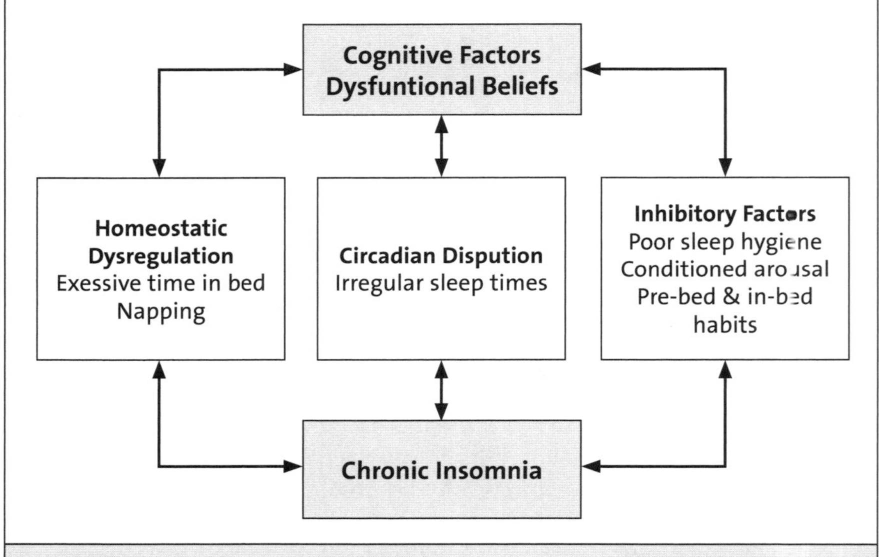

Figure 2
Behavioral, cognitive, and biological interactions leading to chronic insomnia. Reprinted with permission from "Cognitive-Behavioral Therapy for Primary Insomnia," by J. D. Edinger and M. K. Means, 2005, *Clinical Psychology Review, 25*, p. 542. © 2005 by Elsevier

This model provides a perspective that accounts for the various factors that can affect sleep and result in symptoms of insomnia. It presents a static picture that allows a clinician to consider the factors contributing to insomnia symptoms at any given time. In addition, it recognizes that individual differences in homeostatic sleep drive, circadian rhythmicity, and behavioral and cognitive factors can vary across patients. Consequently, the relative contribution of each factor to the presenting symptoms must be considered when conceptualizing treatment and initiating therapy. Further, at any time in the trajectory of insomnia symptoms, these biological, behavioral, and cognitive influences can vary in the magnitude with which they contribute to and maintain the insomnia symptoms. Spielman (1986) formulated a framework that considers the development of insomnia symptoms. While Spielman's framework predates other models of insomnia, it provides a general foundation to account for the progression of insomnia over time. More recent models as described above have filled in the details which support his general framework.

Spielman's organizational framework explaining insomnia distinguishes between factors that precipitate insomnia symptoms and those that perpetuate them, while also recognizing the importance of predisposing vulnerabilities in the development of symptoms (Spielman, 1986). The *3-P Model* presents a tripartite conceptualization for insomnia that incorporates the role of predisposing, precipitating, and perpetuating factors (see Figure 3).

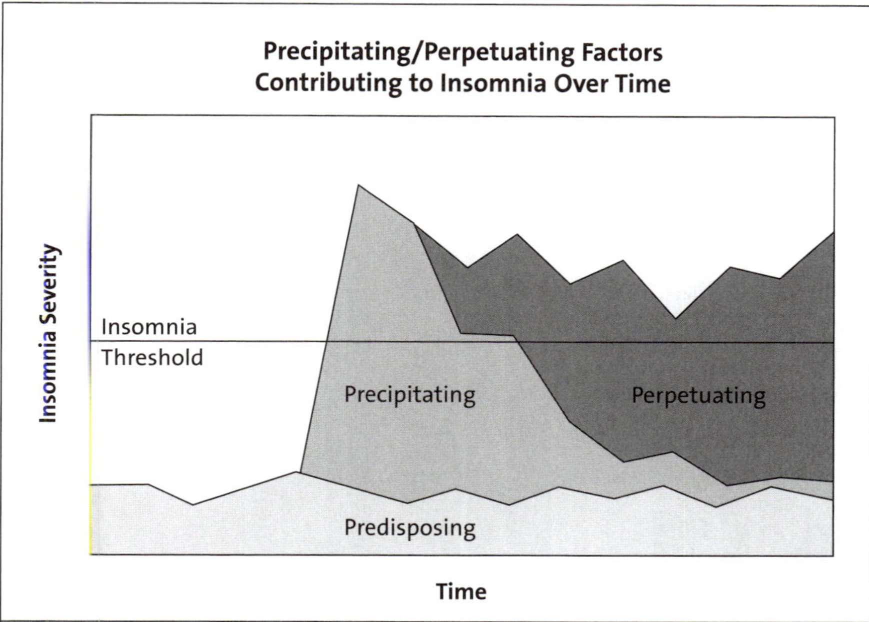

Figure 3
Spielman's 3-P model of insomnia. Reprinted with permission from "Assessment Techniques for Insomnia," by A. J. Spielman, C. Yang, and P. B. Glovinsky, in *Principles and Practice of Sleep Medicine* (5th edition, p. 1634), edited by M. H. Kryger, T. Roth, and W. C. Dement, 2011, St. Louis, MO: Elsevier Books. © 2011 by Elsevier Books

Although predisposing conditions (e.g., impairment in brain areas associated with sleep–wake processes, physiological hyperarousal, anxiety, or coping style) confer a vulnerability to insomnia, they do not necessarily produce significant sleep disturbances unless other conditions are present. In the presence of precipitating circumstances (e.g., significant life events), predisposing conditions can interact with precipitants to produce acute symptoms of insomnia. Predisposing factors are considered necessary but not sufficient to trigger insomnia. With the presence of a precipitant and a predisposing vulnerability, an individual may experience an acute bout of insomnia. In some cases, insomnia symptoms will abate with resolution of the precipitating event.

However, compensatory behaviors (e.g., napping or extending time in bed) meant to alleviate the negative effects of acute insomnia are commonly initiated. Subsequently, even after the precipitating circumstance no longer exists, insomnia symptoms may continue. In such cases, Spielman asserts that perpetuating factors maintain insomnia. Continuing compensatory behaviors meant to alleviate the negative effects of insomnia and conditioning are frequently responsible for the chronic nature of insomnia. Cognitions (e.g., catastrophizing beliefs about the effects of insomnia) can also perpetuate insomnia by increasing the distress and arousal experienced in the anticipation of bedtime.

Spielman's framework serves as a general foundation under which models of insomnia can be evaluated. Models described in this chapter incorporate psychological and biological factors that can function as predisposing conditions or perpetuating factors in the development and maintenance of insomnia. These factors lay the groundwork for effective insomnia interventions.

The neurobiological models described in this chapter support many of the concepts associated with the behavioral and cognitive models. For example, the excess activity observed in brain sleep centers may explain the high-frequency EEG activity described in the neurocognitive model (Perlis et al., 1997) and also serve as the neural foundation for the negatively valenced cognitive activity described by Harvey (2002). While the biological models described may explain the development of insomnia symptoms, the psychological models help to conceptualize how cognitions and behaviors may perpetuate the sleep complaints. Lastly Spielman's conceptual framework serves as the foundation for CBT-I and allows for an integration of biological and psychological models.

3

Diagnosis, Assessment, and Treatment Indications

3.1 Diagnosis of Insomnia

The diagnostic criteria for insomnia have evolved over the past several iterations of the psychiatric (i.e., DSM) and sleep disorder nosologies (i.e., ICSD), and the most recent volumes have introduced a significant simplification in the criteria for insomnia. The current criteria for *insomnia disorder* in the DSM-5 (American Psychiatric Association, 2013) and the ICSD-3 (American Academy of Sleep Medicine, 2014) were developed in parallel so there would be consistency between the nosologies. At the most basic level, the diagnosis of insomnia disorder necessarily requires a subjective complaint of difficulty falling or staying asleep, or of waking up earlier than desired. Mixed insomnia, which is some combination of difficulty falling asleep or staying asleep, or of waking up too early, is the most commonly reported type of insomnia (Morin, LeBlanc, Daley, Gregoire, & Merette, 2006). Isolated sleep-onset insomnia is less common than mixed insomnia. These nighttime symptoms should occur at least three times per week. Insomnia disorder is called persistent if it lasts 3 months or longer, and considered acute if it lasts less than 3 months. Physiological evidence of difficulty sleeping (i.e., a sleep study) is not necessary for an insomnia diagnosis to be made (Littner et al., 2003).

Insomnia can include combined complaints of difficulty falling/ staying asleep or waking up early

Clinical Pearl
When a Sleep Study Is Indicated

It is not uncommon for patients with insomnia to expect that spending the night in the sleep lab to record their sleep would be beneficial for gaining a better understanding of their insomnia. However, an overnight sleep study is not required for a diagnosis of insomnia. Patients come to the clinic complaining about being awake during the night, and a sleep study most likely will confirm that they are awake during the night. Therefore, typically no new information is gained from the sleep study to help with diagnosis and treatment, and conducting a sleep study in patients with insomnia is not an efficient use of sleep center resources. However, if patients do not improve after their insomnia is treated, or if they are at risk for sleep apnea, a sleep study is appropriate. Some patients may be more focused on physical symptoms or have health anxiety and may strongly push for a sleep study, believing that it will reveal the source of the insomnia. Providing information regarding the purpose of a sleep study (e.g., detecting breathing problems during sleep) can be useful with these patients.

The diagnosis of insomnia also requires a complaint of daytime dysfunction

Sufficient opportunity to sleep must be allotted before a diagnosis of insomnia can be considered

Besides the nighttime complaints, the sleep difficulty must cause some daytime distress for the diagnosis to be made. Daytime symptoms commonly include fatigue or sleepiness, difficulty with attention and concentration, irritability, reduced motivation or energy, error proneness, or concerns about or dissatisfaction with sleep. Poor sleepers must also provide themselves with an adequate opportunity for sleep (e.g., reporting that "I'm not sleeping, and I'm tired during the day," would usually justify a diagnosis of insomnia, but if the complaint derives from only allocating 4 hrs for daily sleep, the individual would not be diagnosed with insomnia).

Lastly, a diagnosis of insomnia requires that the sleeping difficulty cannot be adequately explained by another psychiatric, medical, or sleep disorder. Unfortunately, this criterion may not always be clear or straightforward and can require clinical judgment. For example, patients may decline treatment for PTSD because they fear that therapy may reduce their hypervigilance to their environment. From the patient's perspective, while hypervigilance is important for safety, the PTSD symptom (i.e., hypervigilance) is interfering with their ability to fall or stay asleep. In this case, insomnia would not be diagnosed, because the trouble sleeping would be better explained by the psychiatric disorder (i.e., in this case, the PTSD). However, if such patients receive treatment and appreciate symptom relief from PTSD but continue to have trouble sleeping, then insomnia could be diagnosed.

Clinical judgment is important when comorbid conditions exist, to choose best treatment for patient

In depressed patients who also complain of sleep difficulty, deciding to make the diagnosis of insomnia is less clear. For patients with an untreated mood disorder, while the priority will most likely be initiating psychiatric care for that condition, a question arises about whether a comorbid insomnia disorder diagnosis should be considered. In such cases, decisions are best made on a case-by-case basis. If the mood disorder is severe or the patient is in crisis or unstable, depression may better account for the patient's insomnia. However, for a patient with mild or moderate depressive symptoms who is seriously complaining about difficulty staying asleep at night, a comorbid diagnosis of insomnia may be appropriate.

The above definitional changes related to the insomnia disorder represent a significant simplification and consolidation of the diagnostic criteria. In previous editions of both the psychiatric (DSM) and sleep nosologies (ICSD), diagnosticians had a more complicated task of deciding among several insomnia diagnoses. Previous versions of the DSM separated insomnia into primary and secondary subtypes. Primary insomnia was thought to "have a life of its own" with no other primary diagnosis as the cause. Secondary insomnia was thought to be caused by some other primary psychiatric, medical, or sleep disorder diagnosis (e.g., depression, restless legs syndrome, chronic pain); if the primary condition was treated, it was assumed that the insomnia would resolve.

Previous editions of the ICSD, designed by sleep disorder specialists, used a different approach. Several different diagnoses of insomnia were created. Because sleep specialists created this nosology, the diagnoses tended to correspond to theoretical models of insomnia. For example, a diagnosis of *psychophysiological insomnia* from the ICSD would have applied to someone appearing to have cognitive or physiological hyperarousal as the main feature of their sleep difficulty. *Inadequate sleep hygiene* may have been best applied to someone taking daily naps and frequently changing bedtimes and waketimes. *Paradoxical insomnia* may have been the best fit for someone subjectively perceiving no sleep at all for several weeks but appearing only slightly fatigued during the daytime. Within the DSM system, each of these varied insomnia diagnoses would have been called primary insomnia in previous versions of the DSM.

Recent studies of the insomnia diagnoses from the DSM and ICSD have not provided compelling evidence for interrater agreement (Edinger et al., 2011). Because many of the ICSD diagnoses had unacceptably low interrater reliability, the usefulness of the diagnostic system must be questioned.

Besides the unreliability of the DSM and ICSD diagnostic systems, the distinction between primary and secondary insomnia has begun to be questioned. Further, studies have emerged showing that insomnia is an extremely common residual symptom, even after successful treatment, of depression (Nierenberg et al., 2010). In addition, some studies have shown that independent and simultaneous treatment of comorbid insomnia in depressed patients is feasible. These early studies have shown that a better antidepressant treatment response is observed with concomitant treatment, and the insomnia improves (Asnis et al., 1999; Manber et al., 2008; Manber et al., 2016). These findings suggest that the past DSM diagnostic approach of having separate primary and secondary categories may not apply to insomnia disorders.

Some authorities have speculated that the mechanisms that perpetuate insomnia are independent of depression. For example, if poor sleep habits or conditioned arousal develop during an episode of depression, and these insomnia-perpetuating mechanisms are not targeted, even if the depression resolves, insomnia may not improve, and it may be necessary to treat the specific insomnia-perpetuating mechanisms. Similar observations have been made for other psychiatric and medical disorders (Belleville, Cousineau, Levrier, & St-Pierre-Delorme, 2011; Savard & Morin, 2001; Smith, Huang, & Manber, 2005; Zayfert & DeViva, 2004).

3.2 Primary Tools in the Assessment of Insomnia

3.2.1 Clinical Interview

A thorough insomnia clinical interview has many elements

The clinical interview is an important, primary source of clinical information. The interview will be most helpful if it includes the following elements: (a) presenting sleep problem – trouble falling asleep or staying asleep; (b) history and course of the sleep problem – recent onset, intermittent, since childhood; (c) medical history – chronic pain, gastroesophageal reflux disease (GERD), obesity; (d) psychiatric history – depression and/or anxiety; (e) other sleep disorder symptoms – for example, snoring, choking in sleep, restless legs, delayed sleep period; and (f) previous efforts to treat the sleep problem – for example, behavioral therapy, relaxation, sleeping pills. Questions about the sleep setting (quiet, dark, bedpartner snoring) and social environment (relationship stress, newborn in the home) may also help identify impediments to restful sleep. Each of these elements of the interview is described in more detail below.

Presenting Insomnia Complaint

First, patients must report difficulty initiating or maintaining sleep. They may only complain of difficulty falling asleep, but more commonly, patients complain about not staying asleep or a combination of problems of falling and staying asleep. Sometimes patients wake up earlier than they want to and cannot return to sleep. In addition, it is important to identify the duration of these periods of wakefulness. Typically, while falling asleep in less than 30 min is considered normal, most sleep specialist and patients would consider being awake for more than 60 min problematic. It is also important to know the frequency of awakenings during the sleep period (e.g., multiple brief awakenings or one long awakening). Multiple brief awakenings may be a secondary symptom of another sleep disorder such as sleep apnea. Patients should be asked about the daytime impact of their trouble sleeping, as well as whether the daytime symptoms occur only after a bad night. If the symptoms do not depend exclusively on the previous night's sleep, then a comorbid condition may be responsible for the daytime symptoms. For example, persistent daytime fatigue that does not covary with nighttime wakefulness may indicate depression or a medical condition. In such cases, the type of daytime symptoms should be assessed (e.g., fatigue, sleepiness, difficulty with concentration, etc.). For example, while most patients with insomnia report fatigue, irritability, and trouble concentrating, excessive sleepiness (i.e., a significant struggle to stay awake during the day) may signal that another sleep disorder (e.g., sleep apnea) is present. Interestingly, some patients may report laying awake in bed at night for an hour or more and have no complaints. In these cases, insomnia would not be diagnosed, because there is no reported daytime dysfunction.

History of Insomnia Symptoms

The next step in the clinical interview is to learn more about the origin of the sleep difficulty. How long has the patient been experiencing insomnia symptoms? Can the origin be tracked to a specific precipitating event? Some patients are able to track the insomnia to a precipitant, and others are not. Tracking the origin of the sleep problem may help with understanding the specific vulnerabilities to the development of insomnia symptoms. Frequently, the precipitant is a major life event that led to stress and coping problems resulting in poor sleep. For example, a newborn in the house may lead to multiple wake-ups for the parents. In addition, the parents may remain vigilant to the baby's sounds so that assistance can be provided if needed. Someone else may have had a serious medical emergency (e.g., a heart attack that required surgery, a hospital stay, and several months of recovery). Other patients may have endured difficult episodes of depression during which they remained in bed for most of the day for an extended period. Many patients who develop insomnia, in these or other difficult situations, continue to have trouble sleeping for many years after resolution of the original precipitant.

Identifying vulnerabilities may help with future relapse prevention. The chronic nature of insomnia is also useful to understand. Some may experience insomnia symptoms on most nights of the week, while others may have recurrent insomnia, and several bouts may occur during a year, interspersed with periods of normal, consolidated sleep. Some patients will also report having trouble sleeping, for as long as they can remember, and may report that it was well known in their family of origin that they were poor sleepers. Still others will have no clue regarding what precipitated their not sleeping well for years. Finally, the chronicity of the insomnia may also be related to the severity of maladaptive cognitions or behaviors that undermine sleep.

Medical and Psychiatric Comorbidities

Importantly, current medical and psychiatric conditions need to be assessed. Current conditions that interfere with sleep are most relevant. Some commonly occurring conditions include thyroid dysfunction, chronic pain, GERD, frequent need to urinate, asthma, or hot flashes related to menopause. Thyroid problems may cause sleeplessness (hyperthyroidism) or excessive fatigue or sleepiness (hypothyroidism). Chronic pain may cause difficulty falling asleep or restless sleep due to difficulty getting comfortable in bed. Poor sleepers usually have a good sense of how much of their sleep problem is due to the chronic pain (for some, it is a minor impediment, and for others, it is the primary reason for the sleep difficulties). GERD may occur during the night and cause sleep fragmentation. GERD, if left untreated, often is both a precipitant and a perpetuator of insomnia. Frequent urination at night becomes a common problem as people age, and frequent need to urinate may precipitate and perpetuate insomnia. Hot flashes among perimenopausal women are also common and may cause significant difficulty with sleep.

If any of these conditions appear to be less than optimally treated, referral to a physician is warranted. Because numerous medical conditions may interfere with sleep, it is useful to request a medical screening for most insomnia patients, to rule out physical causes for their sleeping difficulties.

Among psychiatric disorders, depression has the strongest association with insomnia. It can be a precursor as well as comorbid symptom of depression (Ford & Kamerow, 1989; Perlis, Giles, Buysse, Tu, & Kupfer, 1997). Additionally, it is the most common residual symptom for those who have recovered from a depressive episode (Nierenberg et al., 2010). Thus, assessment for depression is critical to determine the covariation of the mood and sleep symptoms. Insomnia may occur exclusively or may intensify within a depressive episode, indicating that depression may be causing a symptomatic exacerbation of poor sleep. Difficulty sleeping is also common in those with GAD and PTSD. As with medical disorders, if the psychiatric condition is only partially treated, and residual symptoms of the mood or anxiety disorder remain, optimizing psychiatric therapy should be an important part of treatment planning. Therapy for insomnia may be implemented simultaneously with psychiatric care (Carney et al., 2017; Manber et al., 2016; Taylor & Pruiksma, 2014)

Comorbid Sleep Disorders

Besides medical and psychiatric conditions, symptoms of other sleep disorders should be considered. For example, an evaluation for restless legs syndrome should be conducted when patients complain of uncomfortable or unpleasant sensations in their legs or a strong desire to move their legs, and these sensations are (a) only experienced, or are worse, at nighttime; (b) aggravated at times of inactivity or rest; and (c) relieved when patients move (American Academy of Sleep Medicine, 2014; American Psychiatric Association, 2013).

Often sensations associated with restless legs disrupt sleep onset, as the person feels compelled to move about to relieve the symptoms experienced.

Sleep apnea should be considered when patients report snoring or stopping breathing while sleeping. Insomnia and sleep apnea commonly coexist. It has been estimated that among insomnia patients, 30% have sleep apnea, and among sleep apnea patients, 45% to 50% have insomnia complaints (Luyster et al., 2010). There are several key questions that can help a clinician screen for the possible presence of sleep apnea: (a) inquiries about snoring (e.g., Does the patient have a concern about snoring? Has anyone ever told the patient that they snore loudly? Has anyone ever refused to sleep in the same room with the patient?); (b) asking if anyone has ever observed the patient stop breathing while sleeping; or (c) if the patient has ever awakened gasping for air. Clinicians should consider a referral to a sleep specialist if these signs and symptoms occur in the context of daytime sleepiness or fatigue, obesity, or with a positive medical history for hypertension or other cardiovascular disease (Chung et al., 2008).

In addition, it is helpful to assess the patient's sleep complaints in the context of the *timing* of the sleep period. In instances of circadian misalignment, as observed in *delayed sleep phase syndrome* (DSPS) and *advanced sleep phase syndrome* (ASPS), patients often complain that they either (a) have difficulty falling asleep at a desired time and may not be able to awaken at a desired waketime (DSPS), or (b) wake up too early and cannot fall back asleep during a desired sleep period (ASPS).

To disentangle whether the sleep complaint is associated with a circadian rhythm disorder or a symptom of insomnia requires additional information about the patient's desired versus current sleep schedule. Patients experiencing circadian rhythm disorders often have expectations of when they should sleep that do not match the circadian timing of their sleep period. Patients with these disorders are able to sleep well if they sleep during the times that, biologically, they are predisposed to sleep. For example, patients with DSPS may sleep perfectly well between 3:00 a.m. and 10:00 a.m. on vacation days. However, because of life and work demands, these patients may need to be awake at 6:30 a.m. on most days and, therefore, go to bed at 11:30 p.m., but are unable to fall asleep at this time. These patients then present with complaints of sleep-onset insomnia and daytime sleepiness and/or fatigue. Similarly, patients with ASPS may fall asleep and wake up much earlier than desired, and they may complain of early morning awakenings. In these cases, the sleep difficulty is not due to insomnia, but is secondary to unsuccessful attempts to sleep at times when the circadian and homeostatic drives are not optimal for sleep.

Attempts to Reduce Insomnia Symptoms

Asking patients about previous efforts at treating their insomnia is important because it is common for those who report sleep problems to have tried to solve these problems on their own. Strategies for improvement may include spending more time in bed, taking naps, "trying too hard" to sleep, using caffeine to reduce fatigue, or remaining in bed when not sleeping, so as to "rest." On the surface, these attempts appear logical, but usually these methods will only perpetuate patients' sleep problems.

Finally, if patients have previously consulted a health care professional, you will want to ask about the outcome of that consultation. Also ask if they have used sleeping pills, and were the pills prescription or over-the-counter? Are pills currently being used, and how effective are they? Has a cognitive behavioral or other approach been tried, and how effective was it? If the approach tried was CBT, what aspects of the approach were helpful and in what way? Have other behavioral approaches been tried (e.g., relaxation training)? Some patients arrive for a consultation and express frustration with previous behavioral or other treatments, and claim that they "tried it and it doesn't work." To have the best chance at success, the therapy should be fully implemented (including sleep restriction, stimulus control, psychoeducation, and cognitive therapy) over a sufficient period of time (usually four sessions over 8 weeks is recommended; Edinger, Wohlgemuth, Radtke, Coffman, & Carney, 2007). Patients who inconsistently apply, or actively exclude, components of the treatment will not likely see significant improvement in their sleep. Also, lack of adherence to past treatment, leading to a poor outcome, may discourage patients from making further attempts at any type of treatment, including CBT-I.

External Factors Which Influence Sleep

If any of the sleep symptoms described above are reported in the context of the interview, a referral to a sleep disorders clinic is warranted. But besides screening for potential comorbid sleep disorders, the sleep environment also needs to be evaluated. With respect to ambient room temperature in the sleeping environment, nighttime temperatures that are slightly cooler than comfortable daytime temperatures provide optimal sleeping conditions. However, because of variation in the subjective perception of "optimal," bedpartners may disagree on the best temperature for sleep (Lack, Gradisar, Van Someren, Wright, & Lushington, 2008; Onen, Onen, Bailly, & Parquet, 1994).

Continuous ambient noise during the sleep period can also interfere with sleep, even if habituation to the noise seems to have occurred (e.g., a neighbor's barking dog, bedpartner snoring, television left on). For example, a television that is left on all night, every night, may not seem disruptive to the sleeper, but many brief, unrecognized awakenings may occur and cause sleep fragmentation.

Light is the most important and powerful environmental cue for the timing of sleep. Humans are active in the day and inactive or asleep at night. Our bodies detect the difference between night and day by sensing whether it is light or dark. If we sense light, we are signaled to become alert and active; if there is no light, we are signaled to become quiescent. Blue light in particular is the most potent cue to become alert (Dijk & Archer, 2009). Handheld and other electronic devices (e.g., cellphones, tablets, televisions) provide an abundance of blue light and, when used in the middle of the sleep period, incorrectly signal us to become alert. In general, these devices should be avoided just prior to bedtime and during the night by those with sleep difficulty. Some of these devices can block blue light from being emitted after installation of an app or as a feature of the operating software.

Short Sleepers

Short sleepers sleep < 7–9 hrs but will not endorse daytime difficulties

Occasionally, some patients report that they are not getting enough sleep, and when questioned, it is discovered that they report only sleeping 5 or 6 hrs a night but feel they should be sleeping longer. And yet, some of these patients report no daytime fatigue or sleepiness, have no problems with attention and concentration, are not irritable, suffer no decrements in work or school performance, have not altered their social behavior due to fatigue, and generally have no daytime complaints that are related to their short sleep pattern. In such cases, these individuals are most likely *short sleepers*. Some people require less sleep, and those who are short sleepers would be considered a normal variant and should not be diagnosed with insomnia. Usually these patients present to the clinic because they have been told by a health care professional, or they believe, that they need 8 hrs of sleep. Providing education regarding individual differences in sleep need can often be sufficient to produce relief for short sleepers' sleep concerns.

The information obtained from a clinical interview usually provides clinicians with a wealth of information about the nature and course of the insomnia and associated medical, psychiatric, and sleep conditions. A sample questionnaire to guide an interview that the authors have used is included in Appendix 2 and can be used by readers of this book. The results of a clinical interview are intended to help clinicians prioritize treatment planning. For example, should a referral to a psychiatrist, sleep center, or primary medical care provider be made, or should psychotherapy be initiated for an anxiety or mood disorder? Besides the clinical interview, sleep diaries, and questionnaires that assess symptom severity and maladaptive cognitions can provide additional systematic information about the patient's sleep.

3.2.2 Sleep Diaries

Sleep diaries are considered a gold standard for capturing the subjective sleep experience

While a thorough clinical interview can provide extensive information about a patient's sleep complaints and habits, it primarily yields retrospective information about sleep characteristics, which are subjective reports about sleep quantity and quality. In contrast, sleep diaries provide an opportunity to collect, prospectively, nightly sleep data. Diaries allow a clinician to quantify a variety of sleep indices utilized in the evaluation and treatment of insomnia, and are considered the gold standard for collecting information about insomnia patients' subjective sleep experience (Carney et al., 2012). In fact, this subjective behavioral assessment is a rich source of data regarding individual patients' sleeping patterns. A *consensus* sleep diary has been developed based on the aggregated opinions of many sleep experts (Carney et al., 2012). A modified version of this diary, instructions for completion of the diary, and directions for calculating the necessary sleep indices described below can be found in Appendices 3 and 4. The diaries may be freely used by readers.

Typically, 1 to 2 weeks of a sleep diary will serve as a good baseline indicator of a patient's sleep patterns. These diaries are completed by patients prior to treatment initiation. Diaries are also completed nightly throughout the treatment phase to monitor adherence to treatment recommendations and changes in sleep indices relevant to treatment progress. Information from the sleep diary usually includes bedtime, sleep onset latency (SOL), number of awakenings, length of awakenings, time of final awakening, and out-of-bed time. Finally, a global subjective rating of the quality of the prior night's sleep is obtained from patients. Napping and medication or substance use are also important to collect using the diary and can be added as needed, based on information obtained from the clinical interview.

Data from the diary are used to compute a series of additional sleep indices that are then incorporated into the treatment phase to establish and modify prescriptive recommendations and to evaluate treatment progress. These indices include time in bed (TIB), total sleep time (TST), wake after sleep onset (WASO), and sleep efficiency (SE%). SE% is the ratio of TST to TIB and is multiplied by 100 in order to reflect an estimate of the percentage of the time spent in bed that the patient was asleep. An average TST is calculated from the nightly TST calculations on the baseline diaries. This average TST is used to prescribe the amount of time the patient will be allowed to remain in bed once treatment begins. The average value of SE%, because it serves as a primary measure of sleep consolidation, is monitored during treatment and used to further refine the TIB prescription. Generally, 85% SE% is the treatment target, although it is not uncommon to have SE%s greater than 85% upon treatment completion. For more detailed information about the calculation of each of these quantities consult Appendix 4.

Sleep diaries provide clinicians and researchers with highly specific sleep indices that are utilized to track treatment progress. While these variables are quantifiable and, as such, are useful indicators of treatment change, Morin, Belleville, Bélanger, and Ivers (2011) caution against relying solely on sleep diaries that may not provide sufficient data to comprehensively evaluate the patient's experience of insomnia.

3.2.3 Insomnia Severity Index

The ISI provides information about the magnitude and impact of insomnia symptoms

We recommend the inclusion of the Insomnia Severity Index (ISI) to complement sleep diary data with information about the magnitude and impact of insomnia symptoms. The ISI, originally developed to accurately evaluate outcomes in treatment studies, is a brief, psychometrically sound instrument (Bastien, Vallières, & Morin, 2001). Recent research studies support the use of the ISI in clinical settings to facilitate screening of symptoms and evaluate patients' treatment responses (Morin et al., 2011). The instrument consists of seven items assessed on a 0–4 Likert scale. The seven items evaluate the type of sleep disruption experienced (e.g., sleep-onset insomnia, sleep-maintenance insomnia, early morning awakenings), degree of satisfaction with current sleep, ability of others to discern the impact of the sleep problem on the patient's quality of life, worry or distress about the sleep symptoms, and interference with daily functioning. Scores range from 0 to 28, with higher scores reflecting greater symptom severity. Guidelines for interpreting scores have been provided by Bastien et al. (2001). Scores below 7 are not clinically significant, scores between 8 and 14 suggest subthreshold levels of insomnia, scores 15–21 are associated with moderate insomnia symptom severity, and scores 22–28 reflect a severe level of clinical insomnia. Morin et al. (2011) reported that a reduction in score of $\geq$ 8.4 points is a good indicator of symptom improvement and that a cutoff score of 11 is optimal for an insomnia diagnosis in clinical samples. This cutoff score is associated with 97% sensitivity and 100% specificity in clinical samples. In summary, the ISI is a useful tool in establishing symptom severity at baseline, as well as an indicator of treatment success throughout the course of the intervention and follow-up.

3.2.4 Instruments to Screen for Common Comorbid Psychiatric Conditions

Evaluation of patients presenting for insomnia treatment should be broad enough to encompass, at a minimum, the screening of potential psychiatric conditions that can present as comorbid diagnoses. Although extensive reviews of screening instruments for psychiatric diagnoses that are often comorbid with insomnia and that were described earlier in this chapter (see the section "Medical and Psychiatric Comorbidities") are beyond the scope of this book, recommendations for screening instruments that can be utilized to evaluate the presence of the more commonly co-occurring psychiatric conditions (i.e., MDD and GAD) are briefly discussed here.

The Patient Health Questionnaire-9 (PHQ-9), a psychometrically sound, nine-item scale used to screen for a diagnosis of MDD (Kroenke & Spitzer, 2002) was developed based on the *Diagnostic and Statistical Manual of Mental Disorders,* fourth edition (DSM-IV; American Psychiatric Association, 2000) depression criteria (note: the DSM-5 criteria remain the same). This measure can be used to assess the nine diagnostic criteria in the DSM-5. Each item is rated based on the frequency with which the symptom has been experienced over the preceding 2 weeks (ratings range from *not at all* to *nearly every day*). The instrument provides severity ranges to establish the intensity of depressive symptoms, with scores of 5, 10, 15, and 20 representing *mild, moderate, moderately severe,* and *severe depression,* respectively. The instrument exhibits excellent reliability in addition to demonstrating strong criterion and construct validity (Kroenke, Spitzer, & Williams, 2001). The authors also report that the PHQ-9 has adequate sensitivity and specificity, both reported as 88% when utilizing a score of ≥ 10.

Other self-report or clinician-administered instruments for the assessment of depressive symptomatology that also exhibit strong psychometric properties include the Beck Depression Inventory–II (Beck, Steer, & Brown, 1996), the Center for Epidemiologic Studies–Depression Scale Revised (Radloff, 1977), the Hamilton Rating Scale for Depression (Hamilton, 1960), and the Zung Self-Rated Depression Scale (Zung, 1965), among others.

GAD is the most common anxiety disorder that is comorbid with insomnia. Because worry and anxiety are often reported by patients experiencing insomnia, it is important to screen for the presence of GAD. The Generalized Anxiety Disorder-7 (GAD-7) is a brief instrument which was developed in a manner similar to that for the PHQ-9, for purposes of screening for GAD (Spitzer, Kroenke, Williams, & Löwe, 2006). Although the items do not have a one-to-one correspondence with DSM-5 diagnostic criteria for GAD (nor with DSM-IV criteria, on which it was originally developed), it includes the items that optimize the identification of GAD based on DSM-IV criteria (American Psychiatric Association, 2000). It consists of seven items that are rated on a 4-point Likert scale indicating the frequency with which the symptoms are experienced over a 2-week period, from *not at all* to *nearly every day.* Spitzer et al. identified a score of ≥ 10 as the optimal score for screening for GAD, and scores of 5, 10, and 15 as representing *mild, moderate,* and *severe* levels of symptomatology, respectively. Elevated scores warrant additional evaluation of the patient's anxiety symptoms.

As with the assessment of depression, there are a variety of additional psychometrically sound clinician-administered and self-report instruments that can be used to screen anxiety symptoms. These include the Hamilton Anxiety Rating Scale (Hamilton, 1959), the Generalized Anxiety Disorder Severity Scale (Shear, Belnap, Mazumdar, Houck, & Rollman, 2006), the Beck Anxiety Inventory (Beck & Steer, 1990), the State-Trait Anxiety Inventory (Spielberger, Gorsuch, Lushene, Vagg, & Jacobs, 1983), and the Penn State Worry Questionnaire (Meyer, Miller, Metzger, & Borkovec, 1990). These instruments assess severity of symptoms. However, some (e.g., the Penn State Worry Questionnaire) focus specifically on the unique aspect of worry associated with generalized anxiety symptomatology.

Other less commonly co-occurring disorders may need to be considered during the evaluation of patients with insomnia (e.g., PTSD, bipolar disorder, or psychosis). These or any other disorders will need to be considered based on the clinician's judgment, and may require additional screening questions during the clinical interview.

3.2.5 Instruments to Assess Sleep-Related Cognitions

Assessing sleep-related beliefs informs treatment by identifying thoughts that perpetuate insomnia

Cognitions, or beliefs about sleep – which may develop during an acute period of insomnia or be long-held – may exacerbate both nighttime symptoms and daytime distress. A practical method to systematically learn about patients' cognitions about their sleep is to use an instrument specifically developed for this purpose – for example, the Dysfunctional Beliefs and Attitudes about Sleep Scale (DBAS; Morin, Vallières, & Ivers, 2007). The scale was originally developed with 30 items, but a more recent psychometric analysis has found that a shorter 16-item scale (DBAS-16) provides a reliable and valid assessment of sleep-related cognitions (Morin et al., 2007). Four subscales from the DBAS-16 were extracted using factor analysis: consequences of poor sleep (e.g., "Without an adequate night's sleep, I can hardly function the next day"), worry about poor sleep and feeling helpless (e.g., "I am worried that I may lose control over my abilities to sleep" or "I can't ever predict whether I'll have a good or poor night's sleep"), expectations of sleep needs (e.g., "I need 8 hrs of sleep to feel refreshed and function well during the day"), and medication as a solution (e.g., "Medication is probably the only solution to sleeplessness"). Responses to the items are made on a 10-point Likert scale which ranges from *strongly disagree* to *strongly agree.* Higher total scores indicate that the beliefs are more strongly held, and altering or challenging those cognitions may need to be a focus of the insomnia treatment.

Besides the total score showing the overall strength of cognitions about sleep, consideration of responses to the individual items may point to specific areas of problematic beliefs. These specific beliefs can then be targeted for intervention. For example, if a patient strongly agrees that insomnia "will interfere with my daily activities," and that they "avoid or cancel obligations (social, family) after a poor night's sleep," then focusing specifically on daytime consequences may be useful (e.g., finding examples of adequate functioning even after a poor night's sleep). In summary, the DBAS-16 is a helpful instrument to gain a better understanding of the type and strength of the cognitions that may be perpetuating a patient's insomnia.

Other scales have been developed by sleep experts to assess cognitions that are related to specific aspects of their theoretical model. For example, Harvey (2002) proposed that safety behaviors serve to perpetuate insomnia. Patients who enact safety behaviors do so in attempts to reduce nighttime sleep difficulty and improve daytime functioning after a poor night's sleep. However, engaging in these behaviors may reduce their exposure to disconfirming evidence of inaccurate beliefs. The Sleep-Related Behaviors Questionnaire (SRBQ) was developed to identify which safety behaviors patients with insomnia are using. The scale consists of 32 items that ask the patient to rate how frequently they engage in the behaviors listed "to cope with tiredness or improve your sleep" (e.g., "I try to stop all thinking when trying to get to sleep," or "I take on fewer social commitments," or "I catch up on sleep by napping"). Unfortunately, this questionnaire has not been widely used, and no clinical cutoff scores have been established.

The Glasgow Content of Thoughts Inventory (GCTI; Harvey & Espie, 2004) asks patients to identify specific thoughts (from a list of 25) that they have when lying awake. The items are clustered into three subscales that identify cognitions that focus on (a) rehearsing, planning, or problem solving (e.g., "things the patient may have to do the next day"), (b) sleep and wakefulness (e.g., "how mentally awake the patient feels" or "how bad the patient is at sleeping"), and (c) self-awareness and sensory awareness (e.g., "how tired or sleepy the patientsfeels" or "noises the patient hears"). The scale is to be used to identify thoughts which occur during the night. Clinical cutoff scores are not given for this scale.

3.3 Other Methods of Assessing Sleep: Polysomnography and Actigraphy

Overnight PSG only recommended when other sleep disorders, e.g., sleep apnea, are suspected

The assessment of insomnia typically does not require an overnight sleep study (i.e., PSG). The AASM (Schutte-Rodin et al., 2008) does not recommend PSG for those with insomnia, at least for an initial evaluation, unless another sleep disorder such as sleep apnea is suspected. However, if attempts have been made to improve the patient's poor sleep, and they have adhered to the therapy, but the insomnia seems to be resistant to change, then a sleep study may be warranted. Sleep studies are covered in the US by Medicare and most insurance providers.

A sleep study requires referral to a sleep laboratory, usually for an initial evaluation by a sleep specialist and then spending the night in the lab. During the PSG, a technician attaches numerous sensors to the head and body. These sensors collect physiological information regarding brainwaves, eye movements, muscle tone, airflow from the nose and mouth, oxygen levels in the blood, and breathing effort from the chest. In addition, a video recording is made of the sleep period to capture any nocturnal behaviors. A PSG, by recording brainwaves and eye movements, is the only method for assessing the physiological stages – non–rapid eye movement (non-REM) and REM – of sleep. The most common clinical use of an overnight PSG is to detect whether or not a patient has breathing problems during sleep (i.e., sleep apnea) and the severity of the problem. For patients with insomnia and no other sleep disorder, a sleep study may show that they are awake during their sleep period, but this finding will already be known from the clinical interview and behavioral assessment. Thus, a sleep study for those with insomnia typically does not yield new findings and is typically reserved for nonresponders to treatment.

Actigraphy records body movement and presumes that if no movement occurs, the person is asleep

Another frequently used method of assessment in sleep is actigraphy. Actigraphy does not measure sleep per se, but a correlate of sleep. These devices record activity levels, typically in 1-min epochs. Because sleep is correlated with the absence of movement, it is inferred to be occurring when no movement is recorded. Each minute that the actigraph user has no (or little) movement is recorded as sleep. All of these "sleep" minutes can then be summed to calculate TST, and all of the minutes of "no sleep" can be summed to calculate total waketime.

Several devices have been developed for use in clinical sleep medicine and research. The reliability and validity of these devices have been studied, and scoring algorithms have been developed using PSG as the gold standard. These devices work well in normal sleepers; however, they are less accurate in those with sleep disorders. For example, patients with insomnia who are trying to fall asleep may exhibit behavioral quiescence while remaining awake. The actigraph would incorrectly infer that this person was asleep, since it assumes that the lack of movement is sleep. Alternatively, if someone's body moves throughout the night, but they do not wake up, then the actigraph will record too many "no sleep" periods.

Recently, wrist activity recording devices have become mainstream consumer products. Many of these products are worn 24 hrs a day and provide information to the user about their daily rest–activity cycles (e.g., Fitbit, Apple Watch). These devices have allowed many to get a better understanding of their overall activity levels, and helped to facilitate changes in those levels, if needed. Considering the caveats about the accuracy of actigraphs indicated above, the results regarding the amount of waketime and sleeptime from a consumer-based activity recording device should be interpreted cautiously. A few researchers have determined that these devices do not meet reliability criteria even in nonpatient populations (Lee & Finkelstein, 2015). A general sense of disrupted sleep, but not the precise amount of time awake may be the best use of the output from these devices.

4

Treatment of Insomnia

4.1 Methods of Treatment

4.1.1 Sleep Psychoeducation

Sleep education is an important component of CBT-I

Essential to most treatment approaches presented here is providing a basic understanding about sleep needs, normal changes in sleep that accompany aging, the effects of sleep deprivation, and the role of the sleep drive.

Sleep Needs

The recommendation for 8 hrs of sleep each night is not universal, because sleep needs vary

When queried about personal sleep needs, most patients will automatically respond that they need 8 hrs of sleep nightly. The National Sleep Foundation (2015) has published sleep duration recommendations that cover the lifespan. According to their recommendations, young adults and adults require approximately 7–9 hrs of sleep, while the recommended sleep duration for older adults is between 7 and 8 hrs (Hirshkowitz et al., 2015). However, the authors note that sleep needs can vary for different individuals, with some people needing more or less sleep than that indicated by these recommendations. The critical point to emphasize when addressing this item with a patient is the importance of avoiding preconceived beliefs that 8 hrs is the "magic number." Much more important is the need to determine each patient's required sleep duration based on individual data rather than relying on a recommended average. With this discussion, patients will often raise concerns about how they will be able know what is right for them. The clinician can explain that individual sleep needs are determined based on the amount of time that will allow them to *wake up feeling refreshed.* One of the therapeutic goals is to ascertain this amount of sleep. Through a collaborative process between the clinician and the patient, the initial amount of TIB prescribed is gradually adjusted until the patient reports feeling well-rested. This process is not always straightforward and usually requires several weeks of refining the TIB prescription before this goal is met.

Sleep and the Aging Process

Often patients' sleep quality and quantity expectations are based on sleep experiences from their youth. As we age, however, sleep changes are normal. Specifically, sleep becomes more fragmented, with more arousals and awakenings possible. Moreover, with age, there can be a slight reduction in sleep duration needs as well as a circadian shift toward earlier bedtimes and waketimes. A discussion that explains these normal aging-related changes and addresses related sleep misconceptions can modify unrealistic sleep expectations of patients and will facilitate treatment.

Time Spent in Bed

Individuals with chronic insomnia are frequently distressed by the thought that they are not sleeping enough, worry about the potential negative consequences of sleep loss, and compensate by increasing the time they allocate for sleep. The assumption that they are not sleeping enough is partially reinforced by their extended periods of wakefulness at night. Patients, however, may not understand that the experienced sleep fragmentation can be a result of spending too much time in bed – that is, they may be getting about 7 hrs of sleep, but the consistently extended time that is spent in bed breaks up the 7-hr sleep period across the 8, 9, or 10 hrs they may be lying in bed. This fragmented sleep is commonly perceived as poor-quality sleep. As described above, TIB is gradually adjusted during treatment to facilitate a more consolidated sleep period.

Clinical Pearl
Conditioned Arousal Leading to Poor Sleep

The sleep fragmentation that occurs as a result of extended time in bed often leads to increased distress and anxiety if the patient remains in bed during the periods of wakefulness. This increased arousal can evolve into a conditioned arousal state so that over time, the bed, and even the bedroom, can become associated with wakefulness and arousal. The conditioned arousal can further compound the sleep difficulties that the patient experiences as a result of extended time in bed. In extreme cases, some patients have called this a "bedroom phobia" or come to refer to their bedroom as a "torture chamber." Patients use these descriptions because the powerful association of arousal and wakefulness with the bedroom is in conflict with the desire to sleep, which leads to frustration, anxiety, and anger.

Sleep Drive

Patients with insomnia also routinely focus on the nights they sleep poorly and frequently fail to recognize that, interspersed between poor sleep nights, there are nights of better sleep. It is important for clinicians to explain the body's innate ability to experience a good night's sleep after a couple of bad nights. The concept of the natural (i.e., homeostatic) sleep drive that helps us to sleep after we have been awake for many hours can reinforce this point by illustrating that a good night's sleep will typically follow a couple of poor nights. Sleep diaries completed prior to treatment can facilitate the demonstration of this concept. Furthermore, the buildup of the sleep drive with longer periods of wakefulness should also be addressed in the context of napping, as a daytime nap taken in an attempt to "make up for" the previous night's lost sleep only hinders the body's natural ability to fall asleep at a desired time the following night.

Sleep diaries are useful to demonstrate sleep concepts such as sleep drive

Circadian Rhythm

Our internal clocks play a significant role in our ability to sleep. At night, this internal clock ramps down the alerting signal as we prepare to sleep. In the morning, the clock ramps up and sends out an alerting signal to wake up and begin our day. This decrease in alertness at night and increase in the morning provides a *sleep window,* which is when optimal sleep will occur. Attempting to sleep outside this window (i.e., when the internal clock is sending out a signal to be awake) is difficult and may lead to frustration and anxiety about the inability to sleep. This tension associated with difficulty sleeping may lead to conditioned arousal to the bed, which can then perpetuate sleep disturbance. Furthermore, if bedtimes and waketimes are variable, a consistent internal rhythm may not be well-established, leading to a weakening of the alerting signal. Habits like going to bed early to ensure an adequate opportunity for sleep or sleeping in after a night of poor sleep tend to undermine the normal functioning of the internal clock. The behaviorally induced, less robust alerting signal may lead to more fatigue during the day and more sleeplessness at night. Although most patients have an intuitive understanding of sleep drive (i.e., they know that after a short sleep they will be sleepier), the importance of keeping regular daily rhythms to maintain good sleep is less well understood. Therefore, providing basic education about the influence of the internal clock on sleep timing helps to clarify the importance of getting out of bed at the same time each day.

The influence of the internal clock on sleep can be explained using jet lag as an example

The control of the timing of sleep by the internal clock can usually be understood in the context of jet lag. A mismatch (lag) between one's internal clock and the local time zone defines jet lag. For example, someone with an 11:00 p.m. to 7:00 a.m. sleep schedule on the US East Coast, who flies to the West Coast will, on their first night, feel sleepy at 8:00 p.m., because their internal clock will still be operating on East Coast time, where it is 11:00 p.m. Likewise, this traveler will wake up at 4:00 a.m., because their internal clock will still be set at 7:00 a.m., which is the local time on the East Coast. After a few days of exposure to local West Coast light/dark cycles, which occur 3 hours later than the traveler's internal clock, their biological clock will be reset to the later local time, and the sleep window will once again be 11:00 p.m. to 7:00 a.m.

As with sleep drive, sleep diaries are an excellent tool to use for identifying variable sleep schedules. After describing jet lag and pointing out the variation in bedtimes and waketimes in the sleep diary, patients can better understand how their sleep can become disrupted by creating an analogue of "jet lag" in their own time zone.

Clinical Pearl
Using Clinical Judgement When Providing Psychoeducation

Clinicians need to consider one caveat when explaining the sleep drive and circadian rhythms to patients. These biological concepts may be difficult to comprehend, and the educational level and intellectual and cognitive functioning of patients must be considered, adapting the presentation of this material as necessary. In some instances utilizing simplified language (e.g., describing sleep drive as the body's natural increase in pressure to sleep, which occurs over time, or the circadian rhythm as the body's internal clock which controls, over a 24-hr period, increases and decreases in alertness) can be helpful. In other cases, simply describing the fact that our brains are responsible for our ability to sleep and also to stay alert may be all that can be conveyed. Clinicians will need to use their clinical judgment and, at times, may even choose to omit explanations of these concepts altogether and focus instead on the implementation of behavioral strategies.

4.1.2 Behavioral Strategies

Stimulus Control

Richard Bootzin developed a treatment for insomnia (Bootzin, 1972) based on operant learning theory, which is called *stimulus control*. Bootzin hypothesized that insomnia occurs because the bed and bedroom no longer serve as a stimulus (or cue) for feeling sleepy and falling asleep, but instead serve as a stimulus for being awake and experiencing negative emotions (e.g., frustration, anger, lowered mood). This inability to fall asleep may develop from engaging in behaviors that are incompatible with sleep such as watching television, using a computer or phone, eating, or trying to sleep when experiencing stress. Quite commonly, those with insomnia say that they may have difficulty keeping their eyes open immediately before going to bed (i.e., sleep drive is strong), but when lying in bed, they cannot fall asleep. Some patients may describe their bedroom as a "torture chamber" or say that they have a "bedroom phobia." Clearly, for these individuals, the bed and bedroom have lost their stimulus control for falling asleep.

The goal of this therapy is to help the individual redevelop or strengthen the association of sleepiness and falling asleep with the bed and bedroom. Therefore, the objective is for the bed to begin to serve as a cue for sleep rather than a cue for being awake. This is accomplished by helping those with insomnia develop consistent routines around bedtime by only going to bed when sleepy, using the bed only for sleeping (except for sexual activity or illness), getting out of bed if sleep does not occur rapidly (within 20 minutes), and getting out of bed at a consistent time each day.

The goal of stimulus control is to help patients reassociate sleepiness with their bed

Sleep Restriction

After observing that those with insomnia spend excessively long periods of TIB trying to fulfill their daily sleep needs, Spielman and colleagues developed *sleep restriction therapy* (SRT; Hoelscher & Edinger, 1988; Spielman, Saskin, & Thorpy, 1987). Those who engage in this pattern believe that if they do not meet their daily sleep needs, they will experience negative consequences (e.g., have difficulty functioning during the day or have negative health consequences). These individuals may spend 9–12 hrs in bed to get 8 hrs of sleep. However, allocating more time than needed for sleep typically leads to fragmented, less refreshing, lighter sleep. Additionally, the periods of wakefulness that occur may weaken the association of sleep with the bed and lead to or exacerbate the poor stimulus control described above. The goal of this therapy is to "right size" the amount of time spent in bed so that it better matches the sleep need of the individual. Typically, sleep need is initially determined from a subjective sleep diary, which is recorded by the patient prior to initiation of treatment. This estimate of sleep need serves as a starting point and may be adjusted up or down depending on the therapeutic outcome. The term *sleep restriction* may bother some patients who already believe that they are not getting enough sleep due to their insomnia. A more palatable (and perhaps more accurate) name for some patients might be *time in bed restriction*.

Extended time in bed leads to fragmented sleep

The implementation of SRT begins with a review of the patient's sleep diaries. From this baseline diary the average TST can be calculated by figuring the sleep time for each night and finding the mean for all nights (see Appendix 4

The goal of sleep restriction is to have the patient's TIB better match their sleep need

for details on calculations derived from the sleep diary). The average amount of TST in the patient's sleep diary plus 30 min becomes the starting point for the amount of time the patient will spend in bed. For example, if the average TST is 6 hrs and 45 min, the total amount of TIB would be 7 hrs and 15 min. This initial TIB prescription may be increased or decreased depending on changes in sleep fragmentation during subsequent weeks. The initial focus early in therapy is to reduce the amount of waketime during the night. However, even as waketime is reduced and sleep becomes more consolidated, the patient may not experience relief in daytime symptoms (e.g., fatigue or sleepiness). Therefore, the second focus of this treatment is to increase the amount of TIB so that a sufficient amount of sleep is obtained to relieve daytime symptoms. If sleep is consolidated, and the patient continues to reports daytime symptoms, more TIB is added. However, the reverse may also occur. From a practical perspective, TIB adjustments from session to session are established by reviewing the average SE% calculated from the sleep diaries. If the weekly average SE% is less than 80% then 15 min per night are reduced from the following week's recommended TIB prescription. Alternatively, if SE% is greater than 85%, an additional 15 min per night can be added to the TIB prescription. This process continues until sleep remains consolidated, and the patient is satisfied with their daytime functioning. When these dual therapeutic goals have been met, it is likely that the individual sleep need of the patient will have been determined at this point in the therapy. The specific method for making decisions to change the amount of time spent in bed is described in Appendix 4.

Standardizing the amount of time to spend in bed may be a novel approach to treating insomnia and create anxiety in some patients. Not being able to stay in bed after a poor night's sleep may be a significant change for some patients. For others, reducing time spent in bed may arouse anxiety because they may believe that reducing TIB will necessarily reduce the amount of sleep they will obtain. Adherence may be improved by acknowledging that this treatment is challenging, and that daytime sleepiness will most likely increase during the first several weeks of treatment. Reminding the patient that increased sleepiness is related to a strong sleep drive and that this drive is critical to consolidating sleep, will help the patient to connect the psychoeducational information with their personal experience.

Clinical Pearl
Lower Limit on a TIB Prescription

Sometimes a patient's average TST from the diary is quite low (i.e., 2–3 hrs). It is common for patients with insomnia to subjectively experience being awake when they are actually asleep. A weekly TST average of 2 or 3 hrs is unlikely, and if used for the TIB prescription may lead to significant sleep deprivation. A rule of thumb is to use 6 hrs as a lower limit for the TIB prescription even if the reported TST is less than that. Also, patients should be advised that if they become excessively sleepy, they should not engage in activities that may become dangerous with lapses in attention (e.g., driving).

Sleep Compression

With its goal of reducing time spent in bed, *sleep compression* is similar to sleep restriction therapy (Lichstein, 1988). However, in contrast to the immediate, rapid reduction of TIB used in sleep restriction therapy, sleep compression slowly reduces it until a satisfactory sleep time is determined (Riedel, Lichstein, & Dwyer, 1995; Lichstein, Thomas, & McCurry, 2011). For example, a patient may spend an average of 9 hrs in bed. These 9 hrs may include 6 hrs of sleep and and 3 hrs of wake. Sleep restriction therapy would rapidly reduce this patient's time in bed by 150 min so that the patient is only spending 6 hrs and 30 min in bed. In contrast, sleep compression would slowly reduce the time in bed over a period of weeks. In the above example rather than reducing time in bed by 150 minutes all at once, it may be reduced by 30 minutes each week over a 5-week period. Some patients may find adherence easier using this gentler approach. The evidence for sleep compression is not as extensive as that for sleep restriction; however, it may be useful in those who struggle with the initial sleepiness induced through quick reductions of TIB through sleep restriction therapy.

Sleep compression is a less abrupt reduction of the time spent in bed than sleep restriction therapy

Sleep Hygiene

Optimizing the conditions for sleep from a behavioral and environmental perspective is referred to as *sleep hygiene*. Suggestions for improving sleep hygiene include making sure that the environment is comfortable, including appropriate temperature, reduced ambient light and noise, and making sure the sleeping surface is comfortable. Any of these environmental conditions may disrupt sleep. Limiting amounts and timing of caffeine and alcohol are recommended. Routine exercise is beneficial for sleep and is recommended. However, exercise should not occur within several hours of bedtime because the increase in body temperature during exercise may interfere with sleep onset. Also, it is recommended that patients do not go to bed hungry; a light snack may help facilitate sleep.

Developed by Peter Hauri, these recommendations were originally customized for each individual based on an assessment of their sleep habits (Hauri, 2012). Currently, however, a set of these recommendations is included as a component of CBT-I. These sleep hygiene recommendations are sometimes conflated with stimulus control and sleep restriction interventions; however, sleep hygiene does not directly address the conditioned arousal or the amount of time spent in bed by patients (Stepanski & Wyatt, 2003). The evidence for using sleep hygiene as an independent, efficacious intervention for insomnia is limited and weak, and sleep hygiene is not considered a primary intervention for insomnia (Irish, Kline, Gunn, Buysse, & Hall, 2015).

Sleep hygiene is not synonymous with CBT-I

4.1.3 Cognitive Strategies

Morin (1993) emphasized the contributing role of dysfunctional cognitions in conjunction with maladaptive behaviors in perpetuating insomnia complaints. Sleep-related worry and dysfunctional beliefs can prompt patients to engage in behaviors that may intuitively make sense, but which are counterproductive to sleep (e.g., believing that everyone needs 8 hrs of sleep to function effectively may compel some patients to remain in bed for extended hours to ensure that 8 hrs of sleep are attained). Moreover, these beliefs can undermine treatment by reducing adherence to behavioral treatment recommendations.

Dysfunctional beliefs about sleep may undermine adherence to treatment

The use of Morin's DBAS (Morin et al., 2007) can help clinicians identify patient-specific sleep-related cognitions that can be targeted in treatment. For many patients, the information provided through a psychoeducational component and the reinforcement of this information throughout treatment are sufficient to modify any maladaptive or catastrophizing cognitions they may hold (Edinger et al., 2001).

Cognitive restructuring can also be emphasized when greater attention to specific sleep-related cognitions is required. In Morin's (1993) CBT-I treatment model, the cognitive component emphasized identifying, challenging, and replacing sleep-related maladaptive cognitions. This can be done through more traditional cognitive intervention strategies (e.g., cognitive reframing) in conjunction with the application of self-monitoring procedures such as thought records (Edinger & Carney, 2015).

4.1.4 Cognitive Behavioral Therapy for Insomnia

The overarching goal of *cognitive behavioral therapy for insomnia* (CBT-I) is to improve sleep by minimizing awakenings. It uses combined psychoeducational, cognitive, and behavioral strategies to work toward (1) consolidating sleep and (2) helping patients discover how much sleep they need to feel well-rested during the day. The foci of the behavioral strategies are to reduce conditioned arousal, develop consistent sleep–wake schedules, and optimize the amount of time spent in bed. Cognitive strategies are utilized to help patients develop more realistic expectations about sleep and minimize catastrophic beliefs (e.g., regarding effects of sleep loss on daytime function) that may undermine the behavioral strategies being implemented.

CBT-I is a hybrid, multicomponent therapy that is widely applicable

Hybrid therapies, which are combinations of the aforementioned therapies, evolved in the 1990s. Investigators began to realize that due to the complicated nature of insomnia, sleep difficulties may arise from many different sources. For example, the underlying sleep physiology may become dysregulated, and a person with insomnia may lose their sleep rhythm. This may occur from an inadequate sleep drive (e.g., from taking naps) or unstable circadian pattern (e.g., from frequently changing bedtimes). Others may not have developed problems with sleep physiology (i.e., sleep drive or circadian timing) but instead have developed conditioned arousal to their bed. In such individuals, even though their body is prepared to fall asleep from a physiological perspective, the bed serves as a stimulus for arousal, and this behavioral conditioning interferes with sleep onset or maintenance. Other poor sleepers may have strong beliefs which lead to thoughts or behaviors that are not conducive to sleep. Most individuals with trouble sleeping have some of each of these elements (physiological, behavioral, and cognitive) contributing to their sleep difficulty. The therapies described above when used separately may not address all of the underlying problems associated with sleep. Thus, the therapies were combined with the goal of having a widely applicable treatment that would work for most people with insomnia. That hybrid therapy is what is meant by the term *cognitive behavioral therapy for insomnia* (most commonly referred to as CBT-I). This treatment, as originally developed and tested, is a combination of sleep restriction, stimulus control, and a psychoeducation module.

4.1.5 Cognitive Therapy for Insomnia

Although CBT-I incorporates aspects of cognitive therapy meant to address the role of cognitions in the development and perpetuation of insomnia symptoms, the extent to which cognitive strategies are utilized and the type of cognitive tools that are implemented in treatment can vary considerably. Originally, the cognitive aspects of CBT-I were addressed primarily through the psychoeducation component of the treatment, and in instances where this was not sufficient, via more traditional cognitive therapy strategies meant to target maladaptive cognitions. Although, as described above, the efficacy of CBT-I has been amply demonstrated, not all patients experience a reduction of symptoms with this therapy. Indeed, some patients may respond better to a treatment that focuses greater attention and emphasis on firmly held maladaptive cognitions.

As described in Section 2.3 (Cognitive Models of Insomnia), Harvey (2002) identified in her model the impact of faulty cognitions on sleep disruption. The model describes how sleep troubles precipitate cognitions that selectively focus on the nighttime sleep difficulties and the daytime consequences of disrupted sleep. These cognitions, in turn, can generate increased arousal. Harvey proposes that it is the maladaptive and faulty cognitions in conjunction with safety behaviors (i.e., behaviors that are meant to minimize potential harm such as such as extending TIB to compensate for lost sleep) that contribute to the excessive negative cognitive activity and may result in experiencing perceived, as well as real, sleep and daytime dysfunction.

It is well-established that dysfunctional or maladaptive cognitions are, in fact, often present in individuals with insomnia. Comparisons of insomnia sufferers and normal sleepers reveal that dysfunctional beliefs as assessed by the DBAS can distinguish the two groups (Carney & Edinger, 2006; Ellis, Hampson, & Cropley, 2007; Morin, Stone, Trinkle, Mercer, & Remsberg, 1993). The development of theoretical frameworks to explain cognitions associated with insomnia, in conjunction with supporting empirical evidence linking cognitions to sleep complaints, has fostered an intensive cognitive treatment designed to address the symptoms of insomnia.

Recent developments in therapy for insomnia emphasize treating maladaptive beliefs more directly

Consistent with the Harvey (2002) cognitive model of insomnia, a corresponding approach for the treatment of insomnia targets beliefs and safety behaviors that perpetuate nighttime and daytime symptoms of insomnia (Harvey, 2005). As with other forms of cognitive therapy, the approach utilizes basic cognitive strategies such as Socratic questioning and behavioral experiments to modify thoughts and beliefs. The intervention consists of three phases encompassing 6 to 12 sessions. Phase 1 examines a patient's nighttime and daytime difficulties and, for each, creates an individualized model of the factors that contribute to the sleep and daytime dysfunction. During this phase, the patient is introduced to the basic concepts of cognitive therapy, including understanding the relationships among cognitions, emotions, and behaviors, and how these associations relate to the patient's unique presentation. Phase 2 emphasizes behavioral experiments that allow a patient to disconfirm distorted cognitions (e.g., misperceptions, beliefs, worries). The final phase reviews gains accomplished in therapy and addresses relapse prevention.

Cognitive therapy for insomnia utilizing Harvey's model has shown promise, although the empirical evidence to support its efficacy is still limited.

Harvey, Sharpley, Ree, Stinson, and Clark (2007) have shown that cognitive therapy effectively reduces insomnia symptoms over a 12-month period. Wong, Ree and Lee (2015) showed that cognitive therapy (an adaptation of Harvey's model to a 4-session intervention) delivered after a 4-week module of CBT-I (psychoeducation, sleep restriction, stimulus control, cognitive restructuring, and worry exercises) produced further gains after expected CBT-I improvements in subjective and objective sleep-related measures. These effects were not explained solely by the passage of time, as participants randomized to a 4-week waitlist group who initially received the same CBT-I intervention did not show additional symptom amelioration beyond that produced by CBT-I.

In the only randomized controlled trial to date comparing the unique contributions of cognitive therapy, behavior therapy, and CBT-I, Harvey et al (2014) randomized insomnia patients to one of three 8-week treatment conditions: (a) behavior therapy (BT – i.e., sleep restriction and stimulus control); (b) cognitive therapy (CT – i.e., targeting unhelpful beliefs, sleep-related worry, attentional bias, and sleep misperception in relation to daytime and nighttime impairment, as well as utilizing individualized behavioral experiments); or (c) CBT (integrated components from the behavior and cognitive interventions and individually tailored treatment presentation based on patient symptoms). Although all three treatments were associated with improvement in nighttime and daytime symptomatology, CBT generally produced greater improvement (i.e., response to treatment and remission rates) at termination of treatment and 6-month follow-up as compared with either BT or CT alone. Interestingly, BT produced faster responses than CT, but the improvements for BT were not sustained over time. On the other hand, CT was associated with lower response rates at termination of treatment but greater response rates at a 6-month follow-up. Based on these findings, Harvey et al. (2014) conclude that CBT is a better treatment option than either BT or CT.

More recently, the same authors further explored the outcomes for their CBT vs. BT vs. CT groups by comparing the efficacy of each of these treatments in addressing comorbid anxiety and depressive symptoms (Bélanger et al., 2016). Each treatment group was divided into those with and without psychiatric comorbidity. In the CBT group, the proportion of responders to treatment and of remitters did not depend on psychiatric comorbidity. However, in the BT and CT treatment conditions, the proportions of responders and remitters were smaller in the comorbid subgroups than in the subgroups without comorbidities, suggesting that combined CBT may be more effective at improving insomnia symptoms than separate BT or CT treatment in patients with psychiatric comorbidity.

While the Harvey et al. study and the Bélanger et al. follow-up study provide strong support for the use of combination treatment, it must be emphasized that this is the first randomized controlled trial to deconstruct CBT and evaluate the unique contributions of BT and CT. Moreover, it is the first trial to utilize a cognitive intervention driven by a specific theoretical model. At this point, most studies that have utilized cognitive components have varied with regards to the cognitive strategies selected. Therefore, while these two studies support the efficacy of a cognitive behavioral approach, until more randomized controlled trials are conducted, the specific effective cognitive components remain undetermined.

4.1.6 Mindfulness-Based Interventions in the Treatment of Insomnia

Insomnia experts may integrate mindfulness practices with stimulus control and sleep restriction

Mindfulness-based strategies that focus on maintaining a nonjudgmental attitude and a focus on the present have received attention as treatment approaches that may reduce presleep arousal and improve insomnia symptoms (Lundh, 2005). In contrast to cognitive strategies that focus on examining and altering maladaptive or distressing thoughts, mindfulness strategies emphasize a nonjudgmental and objective focus on thoughts as well as somatic experiences, and encourage the acceptance and letting go of disruptive thoughts and physical sensations. In the context of insomnia, various mindfulness-based approaches have been proposed as treatment strategies. Some investigators have applied general mindfulness-based stress reduction (MBSR) strategies to examine the effects on insomnia symptoms. Others, however, have focused on specifically tailoring mindfulness approaches to the treatment of insomnia. Ong and colleagues developed a mindfulness-based therapy for insomnia (MBT-I) to specifically target sleep-related symptoms (Ong & Sholtes, 2010). The intervention combines stimulus control and sleep restriction practices with mindfulness practices that emphasize increasing awareness of cognitive and physical aspects associated with insomnia. Individuals are taught ways of distinguishing physical and psychological aspects of fatigue and sleepiness, the emotional reactions to sleep disruption, and ways to effectively manage these reactions through the implementation of mindfulness skills such as meditation and acceptance.

Numerous studies have examined the efficacy of MBSR in treating insomnia. In a randomized controlled trial, Gross and colleagues (2011) compared MBSR to hypnotic medication and found that MBSR improved objective and subjective measures of sleep and insomnia severity ratings to a degree comparable to those in the hypnotic medication group. In an effort to understand how mindfulness might improve insomnia symptoms, a subset of participants from this trial was interviewed in focus groups (Hubbling, Reilly-Spong, Kreitzer, & Gross, 2014). In addition to more general benefits of MBSR (e.g., feeling calmer, experiencing less pain), sleep-related improvements noted by group members included being better prepared to cope with episodes of insomnia and feeling less distressed by insomnia symptoms. Furthermore, body scanning, a common practice in mindfulness meditation, was described as a helpful tool for quieting the mind at bedtime and promoting sleep. More recently, studies have shown that mindfulness can improve subjective and objective measures of sleep, either when used alone (Zhang et al., 2015) or after standard CBT-I treatment (Wong et al., 2015).

In a small randomized controlled trial comparing the effects of MBSR and MBT-I, Ong et al. (2014) reported that both treatments produced significant improvements over a control condition in sleep-related objective and subjective outcomes and presleep arousal, at the end of treatment, with effect sizes that were comparable to those for traditional behavioral interventions for insomnia. Remission rates at 6-month follow-up were comparable in both treatment conditions. With regards to insomnia symptom severity, MBT-I was superior to MBSR. Ong et al. suggest that these specific effects of MBT-I may be due to the behavioral components of the treatment, and recommend larger trials to evaluate separately the effects of the behavioral and mindfulness components of MBT-I.

Mindfulness-based approaches hold promise in the treatment of insomnia and may be particularly useful in targeting specific symptoms of insomnia such as cognitive and somatic arousal. However, similar to cognitive therapy, at this time there are limited empirical findings to support independent use of this treatment strategy.

4.2 Mechanisms of Action of CBT-I

4.2.1 Understanding Sleep Physiology

Providing accurate sleep education lays a foundation that facilitates the process of reframing patient expectations and misattributions about sleep and sleep loss. The fundamental knowledge gained through this psychoeducational process also provides a rationale that will help patients more readily accept and adhere to the behavioral treatment components.

4.2.2 Correcting Maladaptive Behaviors

Patients with insomnia often engage in behaviors that are counterproductive to good sleep (e.g., staying in bed longer, taking afternoon naps) because, at face value, they appear to reduce the consequences of lost sleep. Instructing patients to adhere to standard wake times, avoid daytime naps, and restrict the amount of time they spend in bed, are all behavioral strategies that are meant to increase the homeostatic sleep drive and to regulate circadian rhythm. Adhering to these behavioral strategies helps patients to fall asleep and stay asleep more consistently.

4.2.3 Extinguishing Conditioned Arousal

In patients with chronic insomnia the bed and bedroom commonly are associated with hyperarousal and wakefulness. This problem is maintained if patients continue to remain in bed trying to go to sleep or engage in behaviors requiring wakefulness (e.g., watching TV, working on computer).

Stimulus control therapy recommends that patients refrain from any waking behaviors while in bed. This recommendation helps the individual to: (1) extinguish hyperarousal associated with the bed and bedroom and (2) redevelop or strengthen the association of sleepiness and falling asleep with the bed and bedroom. By no longer pairing the bed with wakefulness or negative emotions (by getting out of bed when awake), hyperarousal associated with the bed begins to diminish.

4.2.4 Targeting Maladaptive Cognitions

Sleep-related maladaptive cognitions, such as having unrealistic expectations about sleep, catastrophizing the effects of sleep loss, or selectively attending to bodily sensations, are commonly experienced by insomnia patients. These cognitions can further lead to and exacerbate counterproductive sleep behaviors and hyperarousal. The information that is covered via the psychoeducation component helps to reframe beliefs and attitudes regarding sleep functioning. This information is further reinforced through behavioral enactment derived from an understanding of normal sleep functioning. Psychoeducation combined with the resulting improvement in sleep is often sufficient to help modify many patients' maladaptive cognitions. For others, a more focused examination of daytime and nighttime cognitive processes that perpetuate insomnia symptoms may minimize the impact of cognitions on affective arousal experienced at night and reduce the dependence on maladaptive habits and safety behaviors.

4.3 Efficacy of CBT-I

Several meta-analyses over the past 20 years have been conducted to evaluate the efficacy of behavioral interventions for insomnia. Reviews of behavioral treatments from the mid-1990s focused more on single component therapies and not the multicomponent therapies (Morin, Culbert, & Schwartz, 1994; Murtagh & Greenwood, 1995). These reviews clearly showed that the stimulus control therapy and sleep restriction therapy (as separate treatments) were the most efficacious in reducing time to fall asleep, reducing time awake during the night, and improving subjective sleep quality. However, smaller effects were found for increases in TST. Furthermore, the reviews reported that the effects of relaxation therapies and sleep hygiene as separate treatments for insomnia had smaller effect sizes relative to stimulus control and sleep restriction.

Since investigators began combining cognitive therapy with stimulus control and sleep restriction into the coherent multicomponent CBT-I, several reviews have been completed (Koffel, Koffel, & Gehrman, 2015; Okajima, Komada, & Inoue, 2011; Trauer, Qian, Doyle, Rajaratnam, & Cunnington, 2015). These quantitative reviews all showed that CBT-I has moderate to large effects on insomnia symptoms. The most recent of these reviews combined the results of 19 randomized controlled clinical trials and found that, by the end of treatment, SOL was reduced by 19 min, WASO was reduced by 26 min, and SE% was increased by 10% (Trauer et al., 2015). Furthermore, these improvements were sustained at the 6-month follow-up. TST was marginally improved with a 8-min increase at posttreatment, and greater increases were observed at 6-month follow-up. Overall, this meta-analysis showed that waketime at night (i.e., SOL and WASO) was reduced for the average patient by 45 min following treatment with CBT-I.

Reductions in nighttime wakefulness are comparable between CBT-I and sleeping pills

In addition, the improvements using cognitive behavioral methods are comparable to improvements seen when using sleeping pills (Smith et al., 2002). The improvements in sleep related to CBT-I treatment persist over time, unlike insomnia treated with sleeping pills, where nighttime wakefulness tends to return once the pharmacotherapy is discontinued (Morin, Colecchi, Stone, Sood, & Brink, 1999; Morin, Vallières et al., 2009).

Finally, CBT-I has fewer side effects than sleeping pills. The primary side effect reported during CBT-I is an increase in daytime sleepiness during the early weeks of the intervention (Kyle et al., 2014). Sleeping pills, on the other hand, have many potential side effects (Longo & Johnson, 2000) including tolerance, dependence, withdrawal effects, memory impairment, and complex behaviors while sleeping (e.g., sleepwalking and sleep driving; Hwang, Ni, Chen, Lin, & Liao, 2010). Some research has indicated that risk of mortality increases in those who chronically use sleeping pills (Kripke et al., 1998; Parsaik et al., 2016). In sum, these meta-analytic reviews show that CBT-I is efficacious, durable, and safer than sleeping pills.

The ACP recommends implementing CBT-I prior to prescribing sleeping pills for insomnia

Based on these findings, as well as their own review of the insomnia clinical trial literature, the American College of Physicians (ACP) has recommended that CBT-I should consistently be the first-line treatment for insomnia (Qaseem et al., 2016). They suggest that sleeping pills should only be considered if residual insomnia persists after a course of CBT-I has been completed and patients are informed of the potential side effects of sleeping pills, and agree to proceed with the pharmacological intervention.

4.4 Variations and Combinations of Methods

Many options exist for delivery of CBT-I

The efficacy of CBT-I is well-established, and it is considered the standard treatment for insomnia. The majority of the data to support its effectiveness are based on individual face-to-face treatment. However, concerns about accessibility to trained therapists (Qaseem et al., 2016) and costs associated with treatment (Daley, Morin, LeBlanc, Grégoire, & Savard, 2009) have prompted sleep specialists to develop and evaluate the efficacy of alternative CBT-I delivery modalities. Group CBT-I and self-help strategies (e.g., bibliotherapy, video or audio recordings, Web-based interventions) show promise as alternative modes of delivery.

4.4.1 Self-Help Therapy

Various meta-analyses and systematic reviews have been conducted to evaluate the effects of self-help approaches to treat insomnia. Van Straten and Cuijpers (2009) identified 10 randomized studies that included a self-help treatment approach compared with either waitlist or treatment control groups. Van Straten and Cuijpers defined "self-help" as any treatment that patients could complete independently. The majority of the studies incorporated some form of written materials, with several utilizing video or audio recordings and only one employing a Web-based approach. Small to moderate effects were shown by the interventions in their abilities to improve sleep diary outcome measures and indicators of depression and anxiety. Although the self-help treatments were comparable to the face-to-face treatments included in the analyses, the authors caution against overinterpreting the results from the small number of studies included and suggest that a publication bias may have contributed to the findings.

A more recent meta-analysis, by Ho et al. (2015) included 20 randomized controlled studies (including the 10 studies in the van Straten & Cuijpers meta-analysis) that incorporated self-help approaches (including seven studies with a Web-based component). Interestingly, the authors note that more recent studies of self-help strategies incorporate more components of CBT-I and share more similarities with regards to content. The results generally reflected effects in the moderate to large range on several sleep diary outcome measures at posttreatment, which appear to be maintained at short-term follow-up. As with the van Straten and Cuijpers meta-analysis, the authors caution that the findings are still based on a limited number of studies, with few studies that compare self-help treatment with therapist-facilitated interventions.

Internet-Based CBT-I

Internet-based CBT-I improves sleep of patients, but effects are smaller than face-to-face treatment

With increased accessibility to computers and the Internet as well as the advent of various Internet-based self-help CBT-I programs, the efficacy of computerized self-help strategies is of particular interest. In a meta-analysis of six computer-related intervention studies (of which five utilized Internet-based treatment) that employed CBT-I treatment components, Cheng and Dizon (2012) found small to moderate effects on sleep diary outcome measures and noted that computerized strategies generally have effect sizes that are 20% to 50% smaller than the effect sizes observed in traditional face-to-face CBT-I.

More recently, Zachariae, Lyby, Ritterband, and O'Toole (2016) presented the results of a meta-analysis assessing the efficacy of Internet-based CBT-I in 11 randomized controlled trials. The authors found effect sizes on outcome measures of sleep diary data and insomnia symptom severity that were similar to those for traditional CBT-I. In addition, the effects were maintained at follow-up, which varied by study from 4 to 48 weeks. Similarly, a single-blind randomized clinical trial of a fully automated and interactive Internet CBT-I program showed that at 1-year follow-up, treatment effects were maintained. Almost 70% of the participants who received the CBT-I program were considered treatment responders at 1 year, and 80% of the treatment responders achieved insomnia remission (Ritterband et al., 2017).

Zachariae et al. (2016) conclude that Internet-based CBT-I can serve as an alternative efficacious treatment modality for insomnia, and point out that incorporating personal support during the intervention may enhance the effectiveness of the intervention. Krystal and Prather (2017) caution against premature widespread use of Internet-based CBT-I programs, given the current state of the literature. The majority of studies recruit self-selected individuals who are adept with both computers and an Internet platform; some study samples also suffer from restricted demographic characteristics (e.g., including only highly educated, White participants). Internet-based programs have the potential to reach a large and diverse group of individuals; however, research is needed to explore the efficacy of this treatment modality across a wider segment of the population.

4.4.2 Group CBT-I

As with self-help treatment, group CBT-I may provide improvement in insomnia symptoms via a less intensive delivery modality as compared with individual CBT-I. Koffel et al. (2015) examined the effects of eight randomized controlled trials comparing group CBT-I with control conditions, and found that moderate to large effects were present in various sleep outcome variables, which were maintained at follow-up. In some cases (as in TST and sleep quality), the magnitude of the effect sizes was greater on follow-up assessment, a finding consistent with the findings of meta-analyses that have focused on evaluation of individual CBT-I. The authors suggest that group CBT-I may be a viable option as an effective insomnia treatment.

Swift et al. (2012) presented a psychoeducational workshop format that can serve as an alternative delivery format, building on a group approach. Such a modality has the benefit of increasing the accessibility of insomnia treatment in settings in which resources may be significantly limited. The authors evaluated the efficacy of a 7-hr workshop that incorporated the basic components of CBT-I (including sleep restriction, stimulus control, sleep hygiene, and examination of cognitions, as well as relaxation) and a booster session. Improvements in various sleep outcome measures were observed. Moreover, acceptance of, and satisfaction with, the treatment were very high. This treatment modality allows dissemination of CBT-I to large groups of individuals who may not have considered seeking out specialized treatment or who may not have access to appropriate services.

4.4.3 Stepped-Care Approach

The common thread that weaves through self-help treatment strategies and group therapy is the ability to present CBT-I strategies via less intensive procedures that reduce the demand for trained specialists and that maximize the number of individuals who can benefit from treatment. The concept of a stepped-care approach has been proposed as a way to maximize accessibility to treatment when resources are limited (Espie, 2009; Vincent & Walsh, 2013). These models emphasize initial exposure to CBT-I via procedures that can be disseminated widely (e.g., self-help strategies, online programs), with access to more intense modalities (e.g., group and, ultimately, one-on-one interventions) when treatment response is suboptimal. Ideally a stepped-care approach would begin with treatment that was the "(a) least intrusive, (b) least restrictive, (c) least costly, (d) likely to have a good outcome and (e) appealing to consumers" (Sobell & Sobell, 2003, p. 215). However, currently there are no established guidelines to determine who will benefit from the different treatment modalities available, as this area of research is early in its stages of development. We are unable to identify specific characteristics of patients that may be associated with successful response to specific treatment modalities. Edinger (2009) and Manber, Simpson, and Bootzin (2015) discuss the need for research to answer this challenge, in order to develop strategies that will effectively match patients' needs with appropriate resources.

4.4.4 CBT-I Combined With Sleeping Pills

Numerous clinical trials have shown that sleeping pills are effective for rapidly reducing waketime and increasing TST (Nowell et al., 1997). Most sleeping pills were approved for short-term use (< 4 weeks), and in many cases, once the pills are stopped, the insomnia symptoms return. CBT-I, on the other hand, does not improve sleep rapidly, but instead requires consistent adherence to the behavioral recommendations before improvements are achieved. Usually, this requires several weeks of effort (Edinger et al., 2007). Furthermore, CBT-I does not increase sleep time during treatment. However, unlike sleeping pills, treatment gains made with CBT-I are quite durable (Trauer et al., 2015). It seems sensible that the strengths of each of these interventions (rapid improvement with sleeping pills and durability of CBT-I) could be combined to create a maximally effective intervention. However, the results of the clinical trials testing combined sleeping pills with CBT-I have been equivocal. A few studies (Jacobs, Pace-Schott, Stickgold, & Otto, 2004; Morin et al., 1999) have shown a short-term benefit for the combined therapy early in treatment. However, unlike CBT-I alone, these gains were not sustained, even though CBT-I was part of the treatment. These findings have revealed that combining CBT-I with sleeping pills is more complex than initially thought.

Combining CBT-I and sleeping pills has proved to be complicated

A more recent study by Morin, Vallières et al. (2009), using a combination therapy approach, tested whether or not extending therapy (either sleeping pills or behavioral therapy) from the initial treatment phase to a maintenance phase would be beneficial. Treatment included an acute phase which lasted 6 weeks, with all participants attending 90-min, weekly group therapy sessions. Half of the participants were randomly assigned to additionally receive nightly sleeping pills (zolpidem). Following the acute phase, there was a 6-month, extended phase. Participants randomized to active maintenance treatment during the extended phase had monthly CBT-I sessions to address residual insomnia. Furthermore, during the extended phase, in addition to the monthly CBT-I sessions, some participants were randomized to receive 10 sleeping pills each month, to use only when needed. These investigators found that the best outcomes were obtained in those who received combined CBT-I and sleeping pills during a 6-week acute phase followed by the monthly CBT-I maintenance without pills. Those who extended both CBT-I and sleeping pills fared less well. The authors suggest that receiving CBT-I maintenance, without sleeping pills, allows the participants to consolidate their new strategies for overcoming insomnia. It appears that the extended use of pills may interfere with the efficacy of CBT-I.

Extended us of sleeping pills appears to interfere with CBT-I

Clinical Pearl
Is Melatonin Useful in Treating Insomnia?

Melatonin is a hormone released by the pineal gland during periods of darkness (Abbott, Reid, & Zee, 2017). During daylight hours the amount of melatonin circulating is undetectable; however, as the daylight period ends, the pineal gland begins releasing melatonin. Peak melatonin level is reached a few hours after its release begins and coincides with general sleep-onset time. This fact leads many individuals to mistakenly believe that melatonin can relieve insomnia symptoms.

There are several important points that can be communicated to patients inquiring about the utility of melatonin:

- Little evidence supports the use of melatonin for treating insomnia.
- Increasing the level of melatonin to fall asleep (by taking oral melatonin) when the levels are naturally already at their peak does not increase or enhance the ability to fall asleep.
- Research suggests that melatonin is most effective in treating conditions where there is a mismatch between the time when a person would naturally be falling asleep and the situational or environmental time when the person wishes to fall asleep:
  - Jet lag illustrates this concept. When one travels overseas, there is a period of gradual adjustment before one's sleep–wake schedule matches that of the new destination. Over a period of a few days, exposure to sunlight gradually synchronizes biological functions running on a circadian cycle (including melatonin release) to eventually match the sun–dark cycle of the new location. This process can be accelerated by appropriately timing the intake of melatonin.
  - Melatonin has also been shown to be effective in treating circadian rhythm sleep disorders such as DSPS, a condition in which there is a mismatch between the biological sleep-onset time and the sleep-onset time the individual desires to have (Morgenthaler, Lee-Chiong, et al., 2007).

4.4.5 CBT-I in Patients With Comorbid Medical or Psychiatric Disorders

CBT-I is effective in those with insomnia and comorbid psychiatric or medical condition

The original trials using CBT-I were tested using primary insomnia patients. Usually participants were screened and excluded if they showed evidence of insomnia with any comorbid medical or psychiatric disorders. The success of these studies in demonstrating the efficacy of CBT-I has led to many more studies with patients who have insomnia and a medical or psychiatric disorder. The comorbid conditions include chronic pain, fibromyalgia, cancer, depression, anxiety, and alcohol dependence, among others. A recent meta-analysis of 23 randomized controlled clinical trials of CBT-I in those with comorbid insomnia found that the intervention was effective in reducing insomnia in a clinically meaningful way (Geiger-Brown et al., 2015). The improvements in the sleep parameters for comorbid insomnia were not as large as those found in meta-analyses of those with primary insomnia. As Geiger-Brown et al. (2015) note, the smaller treatment response may be due to the sleep difficulty caused directly by the concurrent medical or psychiatric condition. For example, the intensity of chronic pain may fluctuate, and more intense pain may intermittently interfere with sleep consolidation. Some of the pain's influence on sleep may be unrelated to the treatment targets of CBT-I, and therefore limit the impact of the insomnia treatment. In these cases, an intervention that combines CBT-I with an additional treatment for symptoms of the comorbid condition may be optimal.

One of the most common residual symptoms of remitted depression is insomnia. In the last decade, investigators have become interested in whether an independent treatment for insomnia (during ongoing treatment for depression) could be effective in improving sleep. Furthermore, since insomnia is a known risk factor for subsequent development of depression, it may be possible to reduce the recurrence of depression.

In a pilot study, Manber and colleagues (2008) provided initial evidence that CBT-I reduces insomnia symptoms in depressed patients who are taking an antidepressant. Additionally, the depression remission rates were better in those who received the combined treatment. Although this was a small study, it suggested that augmenting medication for depression with CBT-I improves both sleep and mood more than an antidepressant used alone. A more recent multicenter study in a larger cohort of patients (Manber et al., 2016) using the same intervention model (combining medication for depression and CBT-I vs. medication for depression and behavioral placebo) found that the depression remission rates were similar between the two treatment groups. However, remission from depression in the combined CBT-I and antidepressant group was mediated by improvements in sleep, such that larger improvements with insomnia were related to greater reductions in depression. Improvement in depression was not mediated by improvement in sleep in the control condition. Results from these clinical trials highlight the importance of recognizing and treating insomnia in depressed patients, and using CBT-I as part of the therapy may lead to a better overall outcome.

4.5 Problems in Carrying Out CBT-I

The adherence literature for CBT-I is limited, especially as compared with what is known about adherence in relation to the treatment with continuous positive airway pressure in sleep apnea. To date, dropout rates for CBT-I have been estimated to range between 14% and 40% (Matthews, Arnedt, McCarthy, Cuddihy, & Aloia, 2013). Further, Cvengros, Crawford, Manber, and Ong (2015) suggest that adherence may be less than optimal among many individuals, with reduced adherence to treatment recommendations occurring approximately 2–3 days per week during treatment. Understanding and attending to factors that may influence adherence should be an important part of a clinician's task and may help optimize treatment outcomes.

Studies have identified various factors that may explain reduced adherence and diminished outcomes for CBT-I. Empirically supported individual characteristics related to reduced adherence and treatment outcomes include (a) psychiatric symptoms such as depression and anxiety (Hebert, Vincent, Lewycky, & Walsh, 2010; McChargue et al., 2012; Morgan et al., 2003; Vincent & Hameed, 2003); (b) low self-efficacy, lack of behavioral control, limited expectation of change, and perceived barriers (Hebert et al., 2010; Morgan et al., 2003; Petrov, Lichstein, Huisingh, & Bradley, 2014; Tremblay, Savard, & Ivers, 2009; Vincent, Lewycky, & Finnegan, 2008); and (c) maladaptive cognitions (Cvengros et al., 2015; Tremblay et al., 2009). Specific aspects of an individual's sleep experience, such as reduced sleep quality and diminished SE%, are associated with poor adherence (Petrov et al., 2014). Inconsistent adherence to standard waketime recommendations is negatively related to treatment outcome (Riedel & Lichstein, 2001).

Interestingly, less pretreatment sleepiness as well as greater TST and diminishing sleep disturbances across the course of treatment also appear to predict reduced treatment adherence (McChargue et al., 2012; Petrov et al.,

2014; Vincent et al., 2008). While indicators of better sleep as contributors to nonadherence may appear counterintuitive, some investigators suggest that experiencing any amelioration of symptoms during treatment may create a false sense of improvement that leads to a reduction in motivation and, correspondingly, a premature drop in treatment adherence (McChargue et al., 2012). Finally, social support may also increase adherence (Hebert et al., 2010; Petrov et al., 2014).

Close follow-up early in treatment may improve adherence to CBT-I

Petrov et al. (2014) suggested that poor adherence to some of the more demanding behavioral aspects of CBT-I treatment (e.g., sleep restriction, limitations to time awake spent in bed, standard wake-up time) may signal difficulties engaging in treatment. The authors recommend that clinicians attend more closely to the first few nights of treatment and the patient's reactions to treatment recommendations. Matthews et al. (2013) discuss various explanations that may account for reduced adherence to the behavioral components of CBT-I. Among these is the possibility that patients may consider sleep restriction as counterintuitive to good sleep. In addition, patients' objections to the increased sleepiness they experience initially with treatment and to standard wake-up times that must be adhered to on nonwork days are also proposed as potential factors associated with reduced adherence. Similarly, the difficulty some patients experience in identifying activities they can engage in during delayed bedtimes or during nighttime periods when they are awake is an additional barrier to adherence (Matthews et al., 2013).

Motivational interviewing strategies may be useful for enhancing adherence to CBT-I

Research to identify strategies that can effectively address adherence difficulties is lacking. At a minimum, clinicians should consider thoughtful monitoring and discussion of the potential factors described here, as a way to optimize treatment adherence in the absence of evidence-based approaches to managing adherence difficulties associated with CBT-I. Motivational interviewing (MI) strategies have been shown to be effective across a variety of health settings and conditions (Britt, Hudson, & Blampied, 2004). The central premise behind MI strategies is to interact with a patient in a way that will reduce resistance to treatment. In the field of substance use, MI has been shown to reduce resistance to treatment, increase treatment compliance, reduce dropout rates, and enhance treatment attendance, as well as improve treatment outcomes (Sobell & Sobell, 2003). Specifically, MI strategies encourage the clinician to allow a patient to give voice to their experiences and concerns and to empathize with the client. They also emphasize the use of open-ended questions, utilizing reflective listening, presenting and rolling with patient discrepancies, and eliciting self-motivating strategies (Sobell & Sobell, 2003). While the effectiveness of MI strategies has not been evaluated directly in the treatment of chronic insomnia, the use of these strategies may serve to enhance adherence to CBT-I treatment, particularly in the more demanding behavioral aspects of treatment described above, and perhaps to improve treatment outcomes with nonadherent patients.

4.6 Conclusion

CBT-I is widely accepted and has a strong evidence base for improving sleep disturbances and daytime functioning related to these disturbances. Professional organizations such as the American Academy of Sleep Medicine (AASM) and the American College of Physicians recommend this form of nonpharmacological intervention as a first-line treatment for insomnia. Although superficially this treatment may appear to be simple to implement, an understanding of the underlying biopsychosocial model that explains the development and perpetuation of insomnia symptoms is critical for treatment success.

5

Case Vignette

The following case illustrates the implementation of CBT-I with an individual experiencing chronic insomnia symptoms. It provides information about her history and highlights the areas that should be covered in an initial clinical assessment. Following the history, a summary of each session is provided, and corresponding session excerpts describing some of the common themes that present during treatment are highlighted. This case was recreated from various cases that illustrate the usual course of CBT-I; consistent with American Psychological Association ethical guidelines, identifying information has been changed (American Psychological Association, 2017)

The patient, L.F., a Latina woman in her mid-40s, presented to the clinic with complaints of insomnia that dated back 15 years to the birth of her second child. She reported that since then her sleep has been poor; she noted that she experiences difficulty staying asleep nightly and several times during a month also has difficulty falling asleep.

Psychosocial History

L.F. is a second-generation Cuban-American who was born in Florida. She is in a stable marriage and has two teenage children. She completed a master's degree and is employed fulltime as the director of a large organization. She has worked there for 2 decades with several promotions. She reports having an extensive social support network which includes her husband, family, and friends. She denies illicit substance use. L.F. says that she drinks one to two cups of coffee before noon, but no other caffeinated beverages. She drinks alcohol socially, but never more than two drinks. She denies ever smoking.

History of Presenting Problem

L.F. states that she began experiencing some sleeping difficulties toward the last trimester of her second pregnancy. She states that she would need to go to the bathroom frequently during the night and that it would be difficult for her to return to sleep. She expected her sleep to improve after the birth of her child. After giving birth, however, the difficulties continued and were further exacerbated as a result of her infant's sleep schedule. She reports that her infant was fussy, and that for about the first 6 months, the child would wake up crying several times a night. As with the sleep difficulties she experienced in the last trimester, L.F. found it difficult to return to sleep after the nightly awakenings to attend to the baby. During her maternity leave, she would frequently take naps throughout the day when the baby was sleeping.

However, once she returned to work, she found herself worrying about the impact the lack of sleep would have on her work performance. She also reported remaining hypervigilant to sounds from the baby monitor at night, as she expected the child to wake up. This behavior, she reports, continued for many months after her child began sleeping through the night. She states that she found herself waking up frequently even though the child was not crying, and experiencing significant difficulty returning to sleep. She would find herself thinking about activities scheduled for the next work day and worrying about the impact of the sleep loss on her daytime activities. She states that her sleeping difficulties have remained a significant problem throughout the past 15 years, and she has noticed that they have become worse in the past 2 years coinciding with her last promotion and an increase in job-related responsibilities. Additionally, she finds herself experiencing substantial anxiety in the evenings as bedtime approaches, when she begins to worry about what her sleep will be like.

Since her promotion she has also gained increased flexibility with her time, which she views as a positive change. She notes that on days when she does not have any early morning work events or meetings, she will sleep in and go to work later and stay later and sometimes in the afternoon at work she will take a nap in her office if time permits. She reports that she uses the weekend to catch up on sleep, staying in bed until 9:00 or 10:00 the morning or else going to bed early. She denies currently using sleep aids on a regular basis, although a couple of times a month she will take a hypnotic prescribed by her physician. Additionally, she noted that in the past, after suggestions from friends, she tried to maintain a regular wakeup time and avoid naps. However, she felt that these attempts were not helpful and made her feel more tired.

Medical History

Her medical history is unremarkable; her last physical exam was 4 months ago. She is in good health. The only identified concern she reports is her long-term insomnia symptoms. Seven years ago, her primary care physician prescribed zolpidem. She used it nightly with a good response initially. However, after a few years, the medication “seemed to stop working.” Recently she was prescribed eszopiclone by her physician, but she is concerned about needing to depend on hypnotic medication “for the rest of my life in order to sleep well.” She reports sporadic use of eszopiclone currently, approximately two to three times a month and only when she knows the next day she has an important presentation at work for which she “has to be sharp and clear-headed.” She has been considering using melatonin to help her sleep as she has heard from others that it can help treat insomnia symptoms.

Psychiatric History

She denies any psychiatric history or any current symptoms of depression or anxiety.

Family History

Ms. L.F. reports that her mother experienced bouts of insomnia, but adds that they were "not as bad as mine." No other significant family medical history is noted.

Initial Visit Assessment Data

No symptoms consistent with other sleep disorders were reported during the clinical interview. Scores on measures of depression, anxiety, insomnia, and dysfunctional beliefs were as follows: PHQ-9 and GAD-7 scores were within normal limits; ISI was 23 (severe clinical insomnia); DBAS mean item score was 7.2 (mean item scores above 3.8 are suggestive of significant level of unhelpful beliefs; highest mean score obtained was associated with the expectations subscale; second highest mean score was associated with the worry subscale). At the end of the initial visit, the patient was given instructions to complete sleep diaries during a 2-week period.

First Treatment Session

Sleep Diary Data

Mean TIB = 476 min (TIB range 390–600 min), mean TST = 352 min (TST range 255–430 min), mean SE%) = 74% (SE% range 60–90%); bedtimes ranged from 9:30 p.m. to 1:00 a.m., waketimes ranged from 6:00 a.m. to 8:45 a.m. (see Appendix 4 for a copy of this diary. Note: 2 weeks of diaries is recommended for reliable assessment of baseline sleep parameters; Wohlgemuth, Edinger, Fins, & Sullivan, 1999; however, for this illustration, only 1 week of sleep diary is used).

As described in Chapter 4, the first session of CBT-I primarily emphasized providing education about the normal effects of aging on sleep, individual sleep needs, homeostatic sleep drive (the body's natural increase in pressure to sleep which occurs over time), circadian rhythms (the body's internal clock which controls natural increases and decreases in alertness every 24 hrs), and how behaviors can influence these biological functions. Appendix 5 provides sample language that can be used to explain these concepts.

The use of a sleep diary is critical throughout treatment. Therefore, the calculations of TIB, TST, and SE% need to be completed at the beginning of each session. Additionally, these concepts need to be explained to the patient, as they will be referred to routinely throughout treatment. After calculating the sleep variables from the 2-week sleep diary and reviewing the psychoeducation topics with the patient, a series of behavioral recommendations were reviewed (see Appendix 6). These instructions built on the psychoeducation information that was provided during the session. After reviewing the handout, a determination was made regarding how much time should be spent in bed (see sleep diary calculations; Appendix 4).

In this case, the patient's TIB prescription was 382 min (or rounded to 6 hrs and 30 min). Once the TIB was established, a standard wake-up time was set by the patient, with a corresponding recommended bedtime calculated, based on the wake-up time selected and the TIB calculated. (Note: Bedtime is not set in stone, and it is to be used as a guideline; individuals should not go to bed before the indicated bedtime, but also should not retire to bed at the indicated bedtime unless they are feeling sleepy.) The waketime and bedtime prescriptions were established through a collaborative discussion with the patient. In this particular case, the patient decided to set her standard wake-up time at 6:30 a.m., and she agreed to avoid going to bed before 12:00 midnight. Prior to ending this session, it was important to discuss with the patient any particular barriers that she might anticipate with regards to adhering to the recommendations discussed. In this case, the patient voiced concerns about the efficacy of the treatment, given that she had tried some of these strategies in the past without much success:

Therapist: As we were reviewing some of the strategies on the handout to improve your sleep, I noticed that at times you seemed concerned. What are your thoughts?

Patient: Yes, I'm worried. When we met 2 weeks ago, I mentioned to you that I had tried not napping and waking up at the same time every day, and that didn't work at all for me. Why would they work now?

Therapist: Your concern makes sense and is not unusual. If I recall, you had noted that you tried the standard wake-up time and not napping only for a few days. Many patients voice similar worries after unsuccessfully trying on their own some of the recommended strategies. You can find many of these recommendations on the Internet, in magazines, in self-help books, and many folks who come in for treatment have already attempted to use some of these. What we frequently find is that when they have tried these recommendations they have often tried them inconsistently, maybe for a couple of days at a time, or attempted to utilize only one strategy at a time. By combining all the strategies together, we are targeting the things we talked about earlier – we are trying to strengthen your sleep drive, make your sleep–wake cycle more regular so that you start getting sleepy at the same time every night, and also attempting to reduce the waking associations with your bed and bedroom that have been created inadvertently. Your insomnia symptoms developed gradually, over time, and all these factors – your circadian rhythm, your sleep drive, and the associations to the bedroom – were also altered gradually. By following the instructions daily and consistently over time, you will begin to see that you start to get sleepy at around the same time every night, that it's easier to fall asleep and stay asleep, and that you experience less time awake in the middle of the night. Can you think of anything that might get in the way of you following these guidelines in the next week?

Patient: Not really. I mean, it's going to be a challenge, but I'm willing to give it a try.

Therapist: Great. Now, because we are limiting the amount of time that you spend in bed, you might experience some daytime fatigue and sleepiness. It will be important that you avoid napping during the day even if you experience sleepiness. Remember that the longer you remain awake, the more likely it is that you will feel sleepy at night close to the time we have set as your bedtime. Can you think of anything you might be able to do if you find yourself wanting to take an afternoon nap?

Patient: I guess if I'm at work, I can step out of my office, and talk with some of my coworkers. If I'm at home I can try taking the dog out for a walk. I think this might be the toughest one for me, but I will try my hardest.

Therapist: It's very useful to think ahead through some possible solutions to manage difficulties you may encounter during treatment. You will see the effects of your hard work over the next few weeks. One last item before we wrap up, please remember to continue to complete your sleep diary. As I mentioned in our first meeting, throughout the treatment it will be important to complete the diary each morning. Just like we used the diary today to establish what your time in bed prescription is, we will use the diary each week to modify the prescription accordingly until we establish your optimal sleep time.

Second Treatment Session

Sleep Diary Data

Mean TIB = 435 min (TIB range 390–480 min), mean TST = 360 min (TST range 330–420 min), mean SE% = 82.7% (SE% range 77.5–93.3 %); bedtimes ranged from 11:30 p.m. to 12:00 a.m., waketimes ranged from 6:20 a.m. to 8:00 a.m.

In this session it would be helpful to explore where the patient may have experienced difficulties, and help her troubleshoot through these:

Therapist: How did things go for you this past week?

Patient: You know, I thought I would have had difficulty during the afternoons without being able to take any naps, but I managed to keep myself busy and my mind occupied and, surprisingly, didn't feel as tired as I had expected. Also, I struggled to stay up until my bedtime. I was so sleepy each night before bed, but I really tried to stay up. I have been falling asleep really easily.

Therapist: That's great to hear! Last week we had discussed a couple of ways that you might manage that afternoon sleepiness. Not only were you able to anticipate where you might have difficulties, but you planned a way to manage that was effective for you, and even came up with other strategies during the week to help you. Sometimes that afternoon dip in energy can be countered by engaging in activities that are distracting and activating. It sounds like you were successful in managing with that potential challenge. Also, I am glad to hear that you were able to stay up until your scheduled bedtime. I know it can be quite a struggle, and your efforts will begin to pay off in better sleep. I did notice in the diary that on Saturday and Sunday, you stayed in bed about 1 to 1 and a half hours past your prescribed waketime. Can you share with me what was going on? (Note: Extended periods of TIB are reflected in the average TIB for the week, which in this case was much greater than the recommended TIB established in Session 1.)

Patient: I just wanted to lounge in the bed. I really didn't want to get up that early. My entire family was still sleeping, and I just didn't want to get up. I ended up dozing off and getting up a little later.

Therapist: Ok, there are times when it's tempting to stay in bed longer, especially on a day when you don't have any early morning responsibilities. Why might it be important to keep the same waketime on days off?

Patient: Well, I remember you said that not keeping the same waketimes and bedtimes is like flying to another time zone.

Therapist: That is correct, and that is important, because if you vary your bedtimes and waketimes your internal clock may not be well synchronized and can lead to more sleeplessness at night. Habits like going to bed early or sleeping in can undermine the normal functioning of your internal clock.

Patient: (Laughing) On weekends I should have my husband wake up at the same time I have to wake up.

Therapist: Actually, that might not be a bad idea. Many times bedpartners can provide support by following the same guidelines and sleep–wake schedules. Perhaps it's a discussion worth having with your husband.

Patient: He's always been very supportive and wants me to feel better. It doesn't hurt to ask, right?

Therapist: It sounds like a reasonable option. Let's also brainstorm together alternative ways you might be able to manage those mornings when it might be tempting to stay in bed later.

Note: Review of the sleep diary data also occurs at each session, and adjustments to the TIB prescriptions are made when SE% is greater than 85% – by adding 15 min to the TIB prescription, or SE% is less than 80% – by reducing the TIB prescription by 15 min. In this case, the TIB prescription was maintained at 6 hrs and 30 min. Encouragement to continue following the guidelines and a reminder that gradually she will begin to see changes in her sleep were also provided in this session.

Third Treatment Session

Sleep Diary Data

Mean TIB = 400 min (TIB range 390–455 min), mean TST = 358 min (TST range 335–380 min), mean SE% = 85.1% (SE% range 75.2–91.9%); bedtimes ranged from 11:05 p.m. to 12:10 a.m., waketimes ranged from 6:30 a.m. to 6:40 a.m.

Similar to Session 2, every follow-up session generally begins with a review of the week and the sleep diary. In this instance, the patient had improved her adherence to the TIB prescription, with only one significant deviation, and had generally adhered to the standard waketime. Her SE% was 85%, and thus no change was made to the TIB prescription. When the discussion focused on her bedtimes, it came to light that on one night she had not felt well and had, therefore, gone to bed much earlier. Given that the other bedtimes had been generally close to the prescribed time (within 10–15 min), a conversation ensued simply reviewing the rationale associated with the guidelines about avoiding an earlier bedtime than that prescribed and continuing to stick to the standard wake-up time. While checking on her ability to stick to the standard wake-up time on the weekends, the conversation broadened to include a more general discussion about the beliefs she had endorsed on the DBAS at her initial assessment. This discussion provided evidence that the sleep education module as well as discussions during treatment had helped to modify and reduce the intensity of these beliefs – namely, those associated with her sleep expectations (e.g., after a poor night's sleep needing to take a nap or sleep in longer) and sleep-related worries (e.g., worries over losing control over sleep).

Therapist: As you talk about keeping the standard wake-up time throughout the week, what are your thoughts regarding this guideline? How do you think this guideline and the others you are following are impacting your sleep?

Patient: It seems that doing these things is actually helping me take back control over my sleep. I don't want to jinx it, but I think that my sleep is getting better. What is interesting is how doing the opposite of what I had been doing for so long is actually doing something good. I understand the reason for doing them, but it's still surprising that it's working.

Therapist: As we discussed a few minutes ago when we reviewed this past week's diary, your sleep is, indeed, improving. Your average sleep efficiency this past week is 85%, that's a substantial improvement over the 74% sleep efficiency we calculated when you first started treatment. You say that you don't want to jinx it. I'm curious; on a scale from 0 to 10 where 0 is not at all and 10 is the most possible, to what degree do you believe that what you are doing is changing your sleep?

Patient: About an 8. I can definitely see that the changes I've made are making a difference. I guess I still worry that something else might affect my sleep again, and I'll be back where I started.

Therapist: Let's think through that. Remember that there can be external causes for sleep troubles. Let's say you are experiencing some stress at work that causes you to have a few nights of bad sleep. What does that mean to you?

Patient: Well, it means that I'm going to feel tired during the day, maybe make me less sharp at work.

Therapist: Ok, do you think that you will still be able to get your work done competently? What might be the worst thing that could happen?

Patient: Yeah, if there's one thing I've learned during this treatment is that even if I'm feeling tired during the day I can still do my work. I don't think there would be anything too terrible that would happen. If I make a mistake it wouldn't be the end – not like I would lose my job.

Therapist: OK, and what would you do – in terms of your behaviors – if you have a couple of bad nights as a result of work stress?

Patient: (Pause...) I know what I would've done a few weeks ago. I would've slept in, gone earlier to bed and probably taken a nap whenever the chance arose. I know I can't do those things now. So, I would probably stick to the rules I've been following.

Therapist: Yes, and why would that be helpful?
Patient: Because I don't want to spend time tossing and turning and being awake in bed.
Therapist: So, sleeping in, going to bed before you are sleepy, and taking naps have negative effects on your sleep drive and increase the likelihood that your sleep will be broken up during the night. This then makes you feel more tired the next day and creates a vicious cycle of poor sleep, behaviors that continue to negatively affect the sleep, more bad sleep, and so on....
Patient: Oh yes, and I don't want to go down that road again!

This interchange illustrates how sleep education and the gradual sleep changes during treatment can modify maladaptive beliefs. Explicit discussions that link (either directly or indirectly) a patient's beliefs to what they have learned and to the evidence that has been building through treatment gains can be helpful to refute these beliefs and further reinforce the patient's continued efforts to alter behaviors.

Fourth Treatment Session

Sleep Diary Data

Mean TIB = 404 min (TIB range 395–410 min), mean TST = 364 min (TST range 352–372 min), mean SE% = 89.5% (SE% range 85.9–92.9%); bedtimes ranged from 11:50 p.m. to 12:00 p.m., waketimes ranged from 6:30 a.m. to 6:35 a.m.

The increase in the SE% allowed for an increase in the TIB prescription (mean sleep efficiency greater than 85%). Fifteen minutes were added, and the option of either having a later wake-up time or an earlier bedtime was offered to the patient. She chose to maintain her waketime at 6:30 a.m. and move her bedtime from 12:00 a.m. to 11:45 p.m.

Fifth Treatment Session

Sleep Diary Data

Mean TIB = 405 min (TIB range 400–415 min), mean TST = 390 min (TST range 373–409 min), mean SE% = 92.8% (SE% range 87.2–97.2%); bedtimes ranged from 11:40 p.m. to 12:00 p.m., waketimes ranged from 6:15 a.m. to 6:35 a.m.

Another adjustment in the TIB prescription was made following a continued SE% over 85% (an extension of an additional 15 min for a total of 420 min, or 7 hrs of time in bed). The patient reported that her sleep had improved significantly, corresponding with nightly sleep quality ratings of 4 or 5 on the sleep diary. Score on the ISI (ISI = 8) also indicated significant improvement of symptoms. The sixth session was scheduled for 2 weeks later, and the patient was asked to continue logging her sleep during this period. The possibility of termination of treatment in two sessions was also discussed if improvements continued.

Sixth Treatment Session

Sleep Diary Data

Mean TIB = 420 min (TIB range 410–431 min), mean TST = 385 min (TST range 392–405 min), mean SE% = 91.6% (SE% range 88.9–95.0%); bedtimes ranged from 11:20 p.m. to 11:40 p.m., waketimes ranged from 6:30 a.m. to 6:40 a.m.

The patient reported being satisfied with the improvement in her sleep. She also reported experiencing increased energy during the day. An additional 15 min were added to the TIB prescription. The session also focused on having the patient identify what had stood out most for her during the treatment and what specific aspects of therapy she had found most helpful (e.g., understanding how her habits and behavior patterns were undermining her ability to sleep, gaining confidence in her ability to sleep through the night) and most challenging to manage (e.g., difficulty staying up until scheduled bedtime, sticking to the standard waketime). The final session was scheduled for 3 weeks later, with a request to continue completion of the sleep diaries.

Seventh Treatment Session

Sleep Diary Data

Mean TIB = 435 min (TIB range 420–445 min), mean TST = 395 min (TST range 387–423 min), mean SE% = 90.8% (SE% range 88.1–94.5%); bedtimes ranged from 11:00 p.m. to 11:20 p.m., wake times ranged from 6:20 a.m. to 6:30 a.m. Final ISI score was 3.

With SE% consistently in the high 80s to high 90s during the 3-week period and subjective ratings on the sleep diary primarily 4s and 5s, it was recommended that the patient could consider increasing the TIB prescription by 15 min. The patient noted that she was pleased with the improvements and was fine with the current TIB period. She asked if she could sleep in on some days, which naturally segued into the type of discussion usually covered at termination of treatment.

Therapist: So glad that you asked about sleeping in on weekends; it's a perfect way to discuss where you go from here with regards to your treatment. You might recall that when treatment first began we talked about following the guidelines strictly and without deviations in order to make your response to the treatment as optimal as possible. During this time, you have developed a really good understanding of the mechanisms that can influence your sleep – that is, what can improve your sleep as well as what can negatively impact your sleep. You now have a set of tools at your disposal that allow you to tweak, adjust and even "cheat" a little, because you know what it is that you need to do if you begin to experience your sleep worsening. So if you want to sleep in during the weekend, what might be the consequences of doing so, and what might you do to avoid any negative effects of sleeping in?

Patient: If I sleep late on Saturday and Sunday, I imagine that I will be less likely to be sleepy at my usual bedtime. I can only imagine that I might not be happy on Sunday night as I'm getting ready for the work week and run into trouble trying to fall asleep. I also know that it doesn't do any good to go to bed before I'm sleepy on Sunday night, but if I have to wake up early on Monday I'm going to feel it at work. Right? I guess my options are to grin and bear it on Monday or avoid sleeping in. I guess the important thing for me is that I can decide – maybe sleep in one day of the weekend instead of two, maybe avoid sleeping in too late in the morning, or maybe just feel a little more tired on Monday morning but not give in to the temptation to sleep in or nap.

Therapist: Yes, you can make the decision that you want, as long as you know what the potential consequences are and you also know what to do to avoid extended negative consequences.

At this point, the patient appears to understand the potential effects of continuing to engage in maladaptive habits and, more important, recognizes the role that she can play in limiting the continuation of such behaviors as a way to avoid a relapse. Upon completion of the treatment, patients are encouraged to continue to be mindful of behaviors that may negatively impact their sleep and to keep in mind what they have learned in order to adapt and adjust their behaviors accordingly. As with other treatments, patients can be offered future booster sessions as necessary. Figure 4 summarizes the treatment gains on TST and SE% made over the course of treatment.

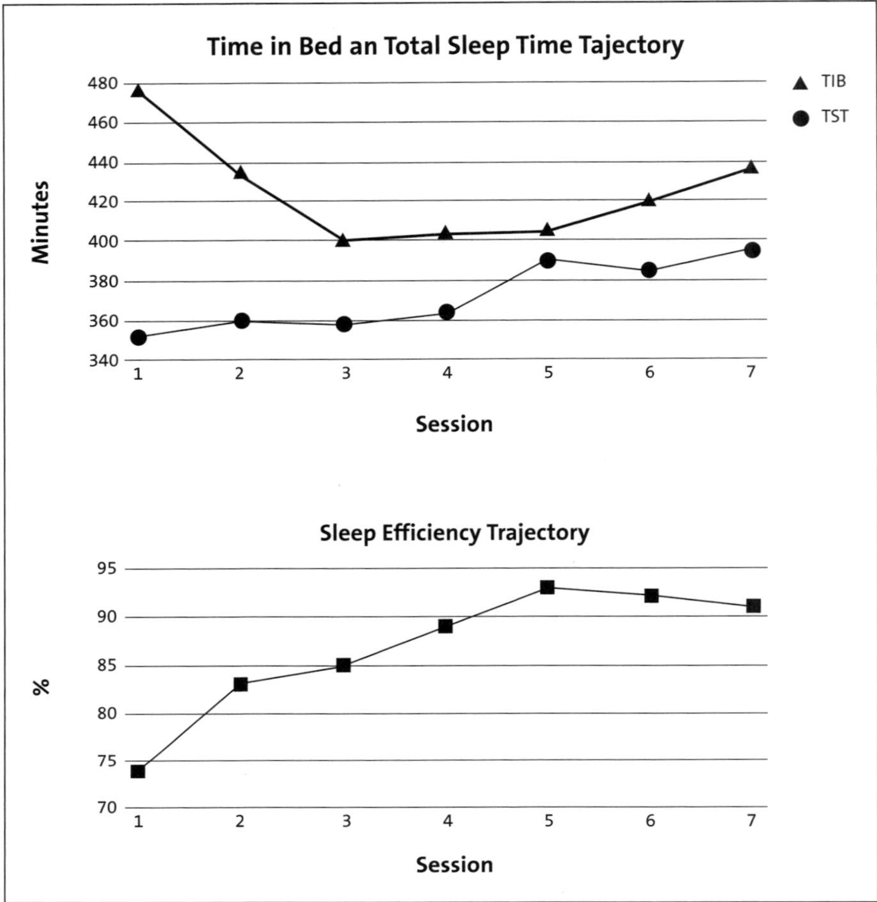

Figure 4
Session-by-session trajectory of total sleep time (TST), time in bed (TIB), and sleep efficiency (SE%) for the patient L.F.

6

Further Reading

Edinger, J. D., Leggett, M. K., Carney, C. E., & Manber, R. (2017). Psychological and behavioral treatments for insomnia: Part II: Implementation and specific populations. In M. H. Kryger, T. Roth, & W. C. Dement (Eds.), *Principles and practice of sleep medicine* (6th ed., pp. 814–831). Philadelphia, PA: Elsevier.
This chapter provides an overview and description of the basic intervention tools used to implement behavioral therapy for insomnia. Also, the various methods for delivering treatment in a variety of clinical populations are described.

Morin, C. M., Davidson, J. R., & Beaulieu-Bonneau, S. (2017). Cognitive behavior therapies for insomnia: Part I: Approaches and efficacy. In M. H. Kryger, T. Roth, & W. C. Dement (Eds.), *Principles and practice of sleep medicine* (6th ed., pp. 804–813). Philadelphia, PA: Elsevier. http://doi.org/10.1016/B978-0-323-24288-2.00085-4
This chapter provides a description of each of the different types of therapies that have been developed for the treatment of insomnia. The evidence for the efficacy and generalizability of these interventions is presented.

Ong, J. C., Arnedt, J. T., & Gehrman, P. R. (2017). Insomnia diagnosis, assessment and evaluation. In M. H. Kryger, T. Roth, & W. C. Dement (Eds.), *Principles and practice of sleep medicine* (6th ed., pp. 785–793). Philadelphia, PA: Elsevier.
A succinct introduction to the assessment and diagnosis of insomnia is provided in this chapter. A number of assessment tools are described, and the usefulness of these tools in helping better understand the presenting sleep problem is discussed.

Perlis, M. L., Aloia, M., & Kuhn, B. (Eds.). (2011). *Behavioral treatments for sleep disorders: A comprehensive primer of behavioral sleep medicine interventions.* Burlington, MA: Academic Press.
This comprehensive book provides treatment descriptions for common sleep disorders. It includes several chapters on various techniques that can be used in the treatment of insomnia.

7

References

Abbott, S., Reid, K., & Zee, P. (2017). Circadian disorders of the sleep-wake cycle. In M. H. Kryger, T. Roth, & W. C. Dement (Eds.), *Principles and practice of sleep medicine* (pp. 414–423). Philadelphia, PA: Elsevier.

Allen, R. P., Picchietti, D. L., Garcia-Borreguero, D., Ondo, W. G., Walters, A. S., Winkelman, J. W., … Lee, H. B., and International Restless Legs Syndrome Study Group. (2014). Restless legs syndrome/Willis–Ekbom disease diagnostic criteria: Updated International Restless Legs Syndrome Study Group (IRLSSG) consensus criteria – history, rationale, description, and significance. *Sleep Medicine, 15*, 860–873.

Allen, R. P., Picchietti, D., Hening, W. A., Trenkwalder, C., Walters, A. S., & Montplaisi, J. (2003). Restless legs syndrome: diagnostic criteria, special considerations, and epidemiology: A report from the restless legs syndrome diagnosis and epidemiology workshop at the National Institutes of Health. *Sleep Medicine, 4*, 101–119.

American Academy of Sleep Medicine. (2014). *International classification of sleep disorders: Diagnostic and coding manual* (3rd ed.). Chicago, IL: Author.

American Psychiatric Association. (2000). *Diagnostic and statistical manual of mental disorders* (4th ed., text rev.). Washington, DC: Author.

American Psychiatric Association. (2013). *Diagnostic and statistical manual of mental disorders* (5th ed.). Washington, DC: American Psychiatric Publishing. http://doi.org/10.1176/appi.books.9780890425596

American Psychological Association. (2017). *Ethical principles of psychologists and code of conduct.* Retrieved from http://www.apa.org/ethics/code/ethics-code-2017.pdf

Asnis, G. M., Chakraburtty, A., DuBoff, E. A., Krystal, A., Londborg, P. D., Rosenberg, R., … Walsh, J. K. (1999). Zolpidem for persistent insomnia in SSRI-treated depressed patients. *Journal of Clinical Psychiatry, 60,* 668–676. http://doi.org/10.4088/JCP.v60n1005

Baglioni, C., Battagliese, G., Feige, B., Spiegelhalder, K., Nissen, C., Voderholzer, U., … Riemann, D. (2011). Insomnia as a predictor of depression: A meta-analytic evaluation of longitudinal epidemiological studies. *Journal of Affective Disorders, 135,* 10–19.

Barion, A., & Zee, P. C. (2007). A clinical approach to circadian rhythm sleep disorders. *Sleep Medicine, 8,* 566–577. http://doi.org/10.1016/j.sleep.2006.11.017

Bastien, C. H., Vallières, A., & Morin, C. M. (2001). Validation of the Insomnia Severity Index as an outcome measure for insomnia research. *Sleep Medicine, 2,* 297–307. http://doi.org/10.1016/S1389-9457(00)00065-4

Beck, A. T., & Steer, R. A. (1990). *Manual for the Beck Anxiety Inventory*. San Antonio, TX: Psychological Corporation.

Beck, A. T., Steer, R. A., & Brown, G. K. (1996). *Manual for the Beck Depression Inventory-II.* San Antonio, TX: Psychological Corporation.

Bélanger, L., Harvey, A. G., Fortier-Brochu, É., Beaulieu-Bonneau, S., Eidelman, P., Talbot, L., … Mérette, C. (2016). Impact of comorbid anxiety and depressive disorders on treatment response to cognitive behavior therapy for insomnia. *Journal of Consulting and Clinical Psychology, 84,* 659–667.

Belleville, G., Cousineau, H., Levrier, K., & St-Pierre-Delorme, M. È. (2011). Meta-analytic review of the impact of cognitive-behavior therapy for insomnia on concomitant anxiety. *Clinical Psychology Review, 31,* 638–652. http://doi.org/10.1016/j.cpr.2011.02.004

Bonnet, M. H., & Arand, D. L. (2010). Hyperarousal and insomnia: State of the science. *Sleep Medicine Reviews, 14,* 9–15. http://doi.org/10.1016/j.smrv.2009.05.002

Bootzin, R. R. (1972). Stimulus control treatment for insomnia. *Proceedings of the 80th Annual Convention of the American Psychological Association, 7,* 395–396.

Borbély, A. A. (1982). A two process model of sleep regulation. *Human Neurobiology, 1,* 195–204.

Breslau, N., Roth, T., Rosenthal, L., & Andreski, P. (1996). Sleep disturbance and psychiatric disorders: a longitudinal epidemiological study of young adults. *Biological Psychiatry, 39,* 411–418. http://doi.org/10.1016/0006-3223(95)00188-3

Britt, E., Hudson, S. M., & Blampied, N. M. (2004). Motivational interviewing in health settings: A review. *Patient Education and Counseling, 53,* 147–155. http://doi.org/10.1016/S0738-3991(03)00141-1

Brower, K. J. (2003). Insomnia, alcoholism and relapse. *Sleep Medicine Reviews, 7,* 523–539. http://doi.org/10.1016/S1087-0792(03)90005-0

Budhiraja, R., Roth, T., Hudgel, D. W., Budhiraja, P., & Drake, C. L. (2011). Prevalence and polysomnographic correlates of insomnia comorbid with medical disorders. *Sleep, 34,* 859–867. http://doi.org/10.5665/SLEEP.1114

Buysse, D. J., Germain, A., Hall, M., Monk, T. H., & Nofzinger, E. A. (2012). A neurobiological model of insomnia. *Drug Discovery Today: Disease Models, 8*(4), 129–137.

Carney, C. E., Buysse, D. J., Ancoli-Israel, S., Edinger, J. D., Krystal, A. D., Lichstein, K. L., & Morin, C. M. (2012). The consensus sleep diary: Standardizing prospective sleep self-monitoring. *Sleep, 35,* 287–302. http://doi.org/10.5665/sleep.1642

Carney, C. E., & Edinger, J. D. (2006). Identifying critical beliefs about sleep in primary insomnia. *Sleep, 29,* 342–350. http://doi.org/10.1093/sleep/29.3.342

Carney, C. E., Edinger, J. D., Kuchibhatla, M., Lachowski, A. M., Bogouslavsky, O., Krystal, A. D., & Shapiro, C. M. (2017). Cognitive behavioral insomnia therapy for those with insomnia and depression: A randomized controlled clinical trial. *Sleep, 40*(4), zsx019.

Carney, C. E., Segal, Z. V., Edinger, J. D., & Krystal, A. D. (2007). A comparison of rates of residual insomnia symptoms following pharmacotherapy or cognitive-behavioral therapy for major depressive disorder. *The Journal of Clinical Psychiatry, 68,* 254–260. http://doi.org/10.4088/JCP.v68n0211

Chang, P. P., Ford, D. E., Mead, L. A., Cooper-Patrick, L., & Klag, M. J. (1997). Insomnia in young men and subsequent depression: The Johns Hopkins Precursors Study. *American Journal of Epidemiology, 146,* 105–114. http://doi.org/10.1093/oxfordjournals.aje.a009241

Cheng, S. K., & Dizon, J. (2012). Computerised cognitive behavioural therapy for insomnia: A systematic review and meta-analysis. *Psychotherapy and Psychosomatics, 81,* 206–216. http://doi.org/10.1159/000335379

Chung, F., Yegneswaran, B., Liao, P., Chung, S. A., Vairavanathan, S., Islam, S., … Shapiro, C. M. (2008). STOP questionnaire: A tool to screen patients for obstructive sleep apnea. *Journal of the American Society of Anesthesiologists, 108,* 812–821. http://doi.org/10.1097/ALN.0b013e31816d83e4

Cvengros, J. A., Crawford, M. R., Manber, R., & Ong, J. C. (2015). The relationship between beliefs about sleep and adherence to behavioral treatment combined with meditation for insomnia. *Behavioral Sleep Medicine, 13,* 52–63. http://doi.org/10.1080/15402002.2013.838767

Daley, M., Morin, C. M., LeBlanc, M., Grégoire, J. P., & Savard, J. (2009). The economic burden of insomnia: Direct and indirect costs for individuals with insomnia syndrome, insomnia symptoms, and good sleepers. *Sleep, 32,* 55–64.

Dijk, D. J., & Archer, S. N. (2009). Light, sleep, and circadian rhythms: Together again. *PLoS Biology, 7*(6), e1000145. http://doi.org/10.1371/journal.pbio.1000145

Edinger, J. D. (2009). Is it time to step up to stepped care with our cognitive-behavioral insomnia therapies? *Sleep, 32,* 1539–1541.

Edinger, J. D., & Carney, C. E. (2015). *Overcoming insomnia: A cognitive-behavioral therapy approach, therapist guide* (2nd ed.). New York, NY: Oxford University Press.

Edinger, J. D., & Means, M. K. (2005). Cognitive-behavioral therapy for primary insomnia. *Clinical Psychology Review, 25,* 539–558. http://doi.org/10.1016/j.cpr.2005.04.003

Edinger, J. D., Wohlgemuth, W. K., Radtke, R. A., Coffman, C. J., & Carney, C. E. (2007). Dose-response effects of cognitive-behavioral insomnia therapy: A randomized clinical trial. *Sleep, 30,* 203–212. http://doi.org/10.1093/sleep/30.2.203

Edinger, J. D., Wohlgemuth, W. K., Radtke, R. A., Marsh, G. R., & Quillian, R. E. (2001). Does cognitive-behavioral insomnia therapy alter dysfunctional beliefs about sleep? *Sleep, 24,* 591–599.

Edinger, J. D., Wyatt, J. K., Stepanski, E. J., Olsen, M. K., Stechuchak, K. M., Carney, C. E., … Radtke, R. A. (2011). Testing the reliability and validity of DSM-IV-TR and ICSD-2 insomnia diagnoses: results of a multitrait-multimethod analysis. *Archives of General Psychiatry, 68,* 992–1002.

Ellis, J., Hampson, S. E., & Cropley, M. (2007). The role of dysfunctional beliefs and attitudes in late-life insomnia. *Journal of Psychosomatic Research, 62,* 81–84. http://doi.org/10.1016/j.jpsychores.2006.06.007

Epstein, L. J., Kristo, D., Strollo, P. J., Jr., Friedman, N., Malhotra, A., Patil, S. P., … Weinstein, M. D. (2009). Adult Obstructive Sleep Apnea Task Force of the American Academy of Sleep Medicine. Clinical guideline for the evaluation, management and long-term care of obstructive sleep apnea in adults. *Journal of Clinical Sleep Medicine, 5,* 263–76.

Espie, C. A. (2009). "Stepped care": A health technology solution for delivering cognitive behavioral therapy as a first line insomnia treatment. *Sleep, 32,* 1549–1558. http://doi.org/10.1093/sleep/32.12.1549

Ford, D. E., & Kamerow, D. B. (1989). Epidemiologic study of sleep disturbances and psychiatric disorders: an opportunity for prevention? *JAMA, 262,* 1479–1484.

Freedman, R. R., & Sattler, H. L. (1982). Physiological and psychological factors in sleep-onset insomnia. *Journal of Abnormal Psychology, 91,* 380–389. http://doi.org/10.1037/0021-843X.91.5.380

Geiger-Brown, J. M., Rogers, V. E., Liu, W., Ludeman, E. M., Downton, K. D., & Diaz-Abad, M. (2015). Cognitive behavioral therapy in persons with comorbid insomnia: A meta-analysis. *Sleep Medicine Reviews, 23,* 54–67. http://doi.org/10.1016/j.smrv.2014.11.007

Glidewell, R. N., Moorcroft, W. H., & Lee-Chiong, T. (2010). Comorbid insomnia: reciprocal relationships and medication management. *Sleep Medicine Clinics, 5,* 627–646. http://doi.org/10.1016/j.jsmc.2010.08.012

Gross, C. R., Kreitzer, M. J., Reilly-Spong, M., Wall, M., Winbush, N. Y., Patterson, R., … Cramer-Bornemann, M. (2011). Mindfulness-based stress reduction versus pharmacotherapy for chronic primary insomnia: A randomized controlled clinical trial. *Explore: The Journal of Science and Healing, 7,* 76–87.

Hamilton, M. (1959). The assessment of anxiety states by rating. *British Journal of Medical Psychology, 32,* 50–55. http://doi.org/10.1111/j.2044-8341.1959.tb00467.x

Hamilton, M. (1960). A rating scale for depression. *Journal of Neurology, Neurosurgery, and Psychiatry, 23,* 56–62. http://doi.org/10.1136/jnnp.23.1.56

Harvey, A. G. (2002). A cognitive model of insomnia. *Behaviour Research and Therapy, 40,* 869–893. http://doi.org/10.1016/S0005-7967(01)00061-4

Harvey, A. G. (2005). A cognitive theory and therapy for chronic insomnia. *Journal of Cognitive Psychotherapy, 19,* 41–59. http://doi.org/10.1891/jcop.19.1.41.66332

Harvey, A. G., Bélanger, L., Talbot, L., Eidelman, P., Beaulieu-Bonneau, S., Fortier-Brochu, É., … Mérette, C. (2014). Comparative efficacy of behavior therapy, cognitive therapy, and cognitive behavior therapy for chronic insomnia: A randomized controlled trial. *Journal of Consulting and Clinical Psychology, 82,* 670–683.

Harvey, A. G., Sharpley, A. L., Ree, M. J., Stinson, K., & Clark, D. M. (2007). An open trial of cognitive therapy for chronic insomnia. *Behaviour Research and Therapy, 45,* 2491–2501. http://doi.org/10.1016/j.brat.2007.04.007

Harvey, K. J., & Espie, C. A. (2004). Development and preliminary validation of the Glasgow Content of Thoughts Inventory (GCTI): A new measure for the assessment of pre-sleep cognitive activity. *British Journal of Clinical Psychology, 43,* 409–420. http://doi.org/10.1348/0144665042388900

Hauri, P. J. (2012). Sleep/wake lifestyle modifications: Sleep hygiene. In J. Blumer, S. W. Lockley & C. H. Schenck (Eds.), *Therapy in sleep medicine* (pp. 151–160). Philadelphia, PA: Elsevier-Saunders.

Hebert, E. A., Vincent, N., Lewycky, S., & Walsh, K. (2010). Attrition and adherence in the online treatment of chronic insomnia. *Behavioral Sleep Medicine, 8,* 141–150. http://doi.org/10.1080/15402002.2010.487457

Hening, W., Walters, A. S., Allen, R. P., Montplaisir, J., Myers, A., & Ferini-Strambi, L. (2004). Impact, diagnosis and treatment of restless legs syndrome (RLS) in a primary care population: The REST (RLS epidemiology, symptoms, and treatment) primary care study. *Sleep Medicine, 5,* 237–246.

Hirshkowitz, M., Whiton, K., Albert, S. M., Alessi, C., Bruni, O., DonCarlos, L., … Kheirandish-Gozal, L. (2015). National Sleep Foundation's updated sleep duration recommendations. *Sleep Health: Journal of the National Sleep Foundation, 1,* 233–243. http://doi.org/10.1016/j.sleh.2015.10.004

Ho, F. Y. Y., Chung, K. F., Yeung, W. F., Ng, T. H., Kwan, K. S., Yung, K. P., & Cheng, S. K. (2015). Self-help cognitive-behavioral therapy for insomnia: A meta-analysis of randomized controlled trials. *Sleep Medicine Reviews, 19,* 17–28. http://doi.org/10.1016/j.smrv.2014.06.010

Hoelscher, T. J., & Edinger, J. D. (1988). Treatment of sleep-maintenance insomnia in older adults: Sleep period reduction, sleep education, and modified stimulus control. *Psychology and Aging, 3,* 258–263. http://doi.org/10.1037/0882-7974.3.3.258

Hubbling, A., Reilly-Spong, M., Kreitzer, M. J., & Gross, C. R. (2014). How mindfulness changed my sleep: Focus groups with chronic insomnia patients. *BMC Complementary and Alternative Medicine, 14,* 50. http://doi.org/10.1186/1472-6882-14-50

Hwang, T. J., Ni, H. C., Chen, H. C., Lin, Y. T., & Liao, S. C. (2010). Risk predictors for hypnosedative-related complex sleep behaviors: a retrospective, cross-sectional pilot study. *Journal of Clinical Psychiatry, 71,* 1331–1335. http://doi.org/10.4088/JCP.09m05083bro

Irish, L. A., Kline, C. E., Gunn, H. E., Buysse, D. J., & Hall, M. H. (2015). The role of sleep hygiene in promoting public health: A review of empirical evidence. *Sleep Medicine Reviews, 22,* 23–36. http://doi.org/10.1016/j.smrv.2014.10.001

Jacobs, G. D., Pace-Schott, E. F., Stickgold, R., & Otto, M. W. (2004). Cognitive behavior therapy and pharmacotherapy for insomnia: A randomized controlled trial and direct comparison. *Archives of Internal Medicine, 164,* 1888–1896. http://doi.org/10.1001/archinte.164.17.1888

Kessler, R. C., Berglund, P. A., Coulouvrat, C., Hajak, G., Roth, T., Shahly, V., … Walsh, J. K. (2011). Insomnia and the performance of US workers: Results from the America insomnia survey. *Sleep, 34,* 1161–1171. http://doi.org/10.5665/SLEEP.1230

Koffel, E. A., Koffel, J. B., & Gehrman, P. R. (2015). A meta-analysis of group cognitive behavioral therapy for insomnia. *Sleep Medicine Reviews, 19,* 6–16. http://doi.org/10.1016/j.smrv.2014.05.001

Kripke, D. F., Klauber, M. R., Wingard, D. L., Fell, R. L., Assmus, J. D., & Garfinkel, L. (1998). Mortality hazard associated with prescription hypnotics. *Biological Psychiatry, 43,* 687–693. http://doi.org/10.1016/S0006-3223(97)00292-8

Kroenke, K., & Spitzer, R. L. (2002). The PHQ-9: A new depression diagnostic and severity measure. *Psychiatric Annals, 32,* 509–515. http://doi.org/10.3928/0048-5713-20020901-06

Kroenke, K., Spitzer, R. L., & Williams, J. B. (2001). The PHQ-9. *Journal of General Internal Medicine, 16,* 606–613. http://doi.org/10.1046/j.1525-1497.2001.016009606.x

Krystal, A. D., Edinger, J. D., Wohlgemuth, W. K., & Marsh, G. R. (2002). NREM sleep EEG frequency spectral correlates of sleep complaints in primary insomnia subtypes. *Sleep, 25,* 630–640.

Krystal, A. D., & Prather, A. A. (2017). Should internet cognitive behavioral therapy for insomnia be the primary treatment option for insomnia? Toward getting more SHUTi. *JAMA Psychiatry, 74,* 15–16. http://doi.org/10.1001/jamapsychiatry.2016.3431

Kyle, S. D., Miller, C. B., Rogers, Z., Siriwardena, A. N., MacMahon, K. M., & Espie, C. A. (2014). Sleep restriction therapy for insomnia is associated with reduced objective total sleep time, increased daytime somnolence, and objectively-impaired vigilance: Implications for the clinical management of insomnia disorder. *Sleep, 37,* 229–237.

Lack, L. C., Gradisar, M., Van Someren, E. J., Wright, H. R., & Lushington, K. (2008). The relationship between insomnia and body temperatures. *Sleep Medicine Reviews, 12,* 307–317. http://doi.org/10.1016/j.smrv.2008.02.003

Lee, J., & Finkelstein, J. (2015). Consumer sleep tracking devices: A critical review. *Digital Healthcare Empowering Europeans: Proceedings of MIE2015, 210,* 458–460.

Li, S. X., Zhang, B., Li, A. M., & Wing, Y. K. (2010). Prevalence and correlates of frequent nightmares: A community-based 2-phase study. *Sleep, 33,* 774–780. http://doi.org/10.1093/sleep/33.6.774

Lichstein, K. L. (1988). Sleep compression treatment of an insomnoid. *Behavior Therapy, 19,* 625–632. http://doi.org/10.1016/S0005-7894(88)80030-3

Lichstein, K. L., Thomas, S. J., McCurry, S. M. (2011). Sleep compression. In M. Perlis, M. Aloia, & B. Kuhn (Eds.), *Behavioral treatments for sleep disorders* (pp. 55–60). Boston, MA: Elsevier. http://doi.org/10.1016/B978-0-12-381522-4.00005-5

Littner, M., Hirshkowitz, M., Kramer, M., Kapen, S., Anderson, W. M., Bailey, D., … Loube, D. I. (2003). Practice parameters for using polysomnography to evaluate insomnia: An update. *Sleep, 26,* 754–760. http://doi.org/10.1093/sleep/26.6.754

Longo, L. P., & Johnson, B. (2000). Addiction: Part I: Benzodiazepines-side effects, abuse risk and alternatives. *American Family Physician, 61,* 2121–2128.

Lundh, L. G. (2005). The role of acceptance and mindfulness in the treatment of insomnia. *Journal of Cognitive Psychotherapy, 19,* 29–39. http://doi.org/10.1891/jcop.19.1.29.66331

Luyster, F. S., Buysse, D. J., & Strollo, P. J., Jr. (2010). Comorbid insomnia and obstructive sleep apnea: Challenges for clinical practice and research. *Journal of Clinical Sleep Medicine, 6,* 196–204.

Mahowald, M. W., Bornemann, M. C., & Schenck, C. H. (2004). Parasomnias. *Seminars in Neurology, 24,* 283–292. http://doi.org/10.1055/s-2004-835064

Manber, R., Buysse, D. J., Edinger, J., Krystal, A., Luther, J. F., Wisniewski, S. R., … Thase, M. E. (2016). Efficacy of cognitive-behavioral therapy for insomnia combined with antidepressant pharmacotherapy in patients with comorbid depression and insomnia: A randomized controlled trial. *Journal of Clinical Psychiatry, 77,* e1316–e1323.

Manber, R., Edinger, J. D., Gress, J. L., San Pedro-Salcedo, M. G., Kuo, T. F., & Kalista, T. (2008). Cognitive behavioral therapy for insomnia enhances depression outcome in patients with comorbid major depressive disorder and insomnia. *Sleep, 31,* 489–495. http://doi.org/10.1093/sleep/31.4.489

Manber, R., Simpson, N. S., & Bootzin, R. R. (2015). A step towards stepped care: Delivery of CBT-I with reduced clinician time. *Sleep Medicine Reviews, 19,* 3–5. http://doi.org/10.1016/j.smrv.2014.09.003

Matthews, E. E., Arnedt, J. T., McCarthy, M. S., Cuddihy, L. J., & Aloia, M. S. (2013). Adherence to cognitive behavioral therapy for insomnia: A systematic review. *Sleep Medicine Reviews, 17,* 453–464. http://doi.org/10.1016/j.smrv.2013.01.001

McChargue, D. E., Sankaranarayanan, J., Visovsky, C. G., Matthews, E. E., Highland, K. B., & Berger, A. M. (2012). Predictors of adherence to a behavioral therapy sleep intervention during breast cancer chemotherapy. *Supportive Care in Cancer, 20,* 245–252. http://doi.org/10.1007/s00520-010-1060-1

Mellman, T. A. (2006). Sleep and anxiety disorders. *Psychiatric Clinics, 29,* 1047–1058. http://doi.org/10.1016/j.psc.2006.08.005

Mendelson, W. B. (1995). Long-term follow-up of chronic insomnia. *Sleep, 18,* 698–701. http://doi.org/10.1093/sleep/18.8.698

Meyer, T. J., Miller, M. L., Metzger, R. L., & Borkovec, T. D. (1990). Development and validation of the Penn State Worry Questionnaire. *Behaviour Research and Therapy, 28,* 487–495. http://doi.org/10.1016/0005-7967(90)90135-6

Monroe, L. J. (1967). Psychological and physiological differences between good and poor sleepers. *Journal of Abnormal Psychology, 72,* 255–264. http://doi.org/10.1037/h0024563

Morgan, K., Dixon, S., Mathers, N., Thompson, J., & Tomeny, M. (2003). Psychological treatment for insomnia in the management of long-term hypnotic drug use: A pragmatic randomised controlled trial. *British Journal of General Practice, 53,* 923–928.

Morgenthaler, T. I., Kapur, V. K., Brown, T., Swick, T. J., Alessi, C., Aurora, R. N., … Owens, J. (2007). Practice parameters for the treatment of narcolepsy and other hypersomnias of central origin. *Sleep, 30,* 1705–1711. http://doi.org/10.1093/sleep/30.12.1705

Morgenthaler, T. I., Lee-Chiong, T., Alessi, C., Friedman, L., Aurora, R. N., Boehlecke, B., … Owens, J. (2007). Practice parameters for the clinical evaluation and treatment of circadian rhythm sleep disorders. *Sleep, 30,* 1445–1459. http://doi.org/10.1093/sleep/30.11.1445

Morin, C. M. (1993). *Insomnia: Psychological assessment and management*. New York, NY: Guilford Press.

Morin, C. M., Bélanger, L., LeBlanc, M., Ivers, H., Savard, J., Espie, C. A., … Grégoire, J. P. (2009). The natural history of insomnia: A population-based 3-year longitudinal study. *Archives of Internal Medicine, 169,* 447–453. http://doi.org/10.1001/archinternmed.2008.610

Morin, C. M., Belleville, G., Bélanger, L., & Ivers, H. (2011). The Insomnia Severity Index: Psychometric indicators to detect insomnia cases and evaluate treatment response. *Sleep, 34,* 601–608. http://doi.org/10.1093/sleep/34.5.601

Morin, C. M., Colecchi, C., Stone, J., Sood, R., & Brink, D. (1999). Behavioral and pharmacological therapies for late-life insomnia: A randomized controlled trial. *JAMA, 281,* 991–999. http://doi.org/10.1001/jama.281.11.991

Morin, C. M., Culbert, J. P., & Schwartz, S. M. (1994). Nonpharmacological interventions for insomnia. *American Journal of Psychiatry, 151,* 1172–1180. http://doi.org/10.1176/ajp.151.8.1172

Morin, C. M., & Jarrin, D. C. (2013a). Epidemiology of insomnia: Prevalence, course, risk factors, and public health burden. *Sleep Medicine Clinics, 8*(3), 281–297. http://doi.org/10.1016/j.jsmc.2013.05.002

Morin, C. M., & Jarrin, D. C. (2013b). Insomnia and healthcare-seeking behaviors: Impact of case definitions, comorbidity, sociodemographic, and cultural factors. *Sleep Medicine, 14,* 808–809. http://doi.org/10.1016/j.sleep.2013.05.003

Morin, C. M., LeBlanc, M., Daley, M., Gregoire, J. P., & Merette, C. (2006). Epidemiology of insomnia: Prevalence, self-help treatments, consultations, and determinants of help-seeking behaviors. *Sleep Medicine, 7,* 123–130. http://doi.org/10.1016/j.sleep.2005.08.008

Morin, C. M., Stone, J., Trinkle, D., Mercer, J., & Remsberg, S. (1993). Dysfunctional beliefs and attitudes about sleep among older adults with and without insomnia complaints. *Psychology and Aging, 8,* 463–467. http://doi.org/10.1037/0882-7974.8.3.463

Morin, C. M., Vallières, A., Guay, B., Ivers, H., Savard, J., Mérette, C., … Baillargeon, L. (2009). Cognitive behavioral therapy, singly and combined with medication, for persistent insomnia: A randomized controlled trial. *JAMA, 301,* 2005–2015. http://doi.org/10.1001/jama.2009.682

Morin, C. M., Vallières, A., & Ivers, H. (2007). Dysfunctional beliefs and attitudes about sleep (DBAS): Validation of a brief version (DBAS-16). *Sleep, 30,* 1547–1554. http://doi.org/10.1093/sleep/30.11.1547

Morris, M., Lack, L., & Dawson, D. (1990). Sleep-onset insomniacs have delayed temperature rhythms. *Sleep, 13,* 1–14. http://doi.org/10.1093/sleep/13.1.1

Murtagh, D. R., & Greenwood, K. M. (1995). Identifying effective psychological treatments for insomnia: A meta-analysis. *Journal of Consulting and Clinical Psychology, 63,* 79–89. http://doi.org/10.1037/0022-006X.63.1.79

National Sleep Foundation. (2015, February 2). *National Sleep Foundation recommends new sleep times* [Press release]. Retrieved from https://sleepfoundation.org/press-release/national-sleep-foundation-recommends-new-sleep-times

Nierenberg, A. A., Husain, M. M., Trivedi, M. H., Fava, M., Warden, D., Wisniewski, S. R., … Rush, A. J. (2010). Residual symptoms after remission of major depressive disorder with citalopram and risk of relapse: A STAR*D report. *Psychological Medicine, 40,* 41–50. http://doi.org/10.1017/S0033291709006011

Nowell, P. D., Mazumdar, S., Buysse, D. J., Dew, M. A., Reynolds, C. F., & Kupfer, D. J. (1997). Benzodiazepines and zolpidem for chronic insomnia: A meta-analysis of treatment efficacy. *JAMA, 278,* 2170–2177. http://doi.org/10.1001/jama.1997.03550240060035

Ohayon, M. M. (2002). Epidemiology of insomnia: What we know and what we still need to learn. *Sleep Medicine Reviews, 6,* 97–111. http://doi.org/10.1053/smrv.2002.0186

Ohayon, M. M., Caulet, M., & Lemoine, P. (1998). Comorbidity of mental and insomnia disorders in the general population. *Comprehensive Psychiatry, 39,* 185–197. http://doi.org/10.1016/S0010-440X(98)90059-1

Ohayon, M. M., Mahowald, M. W., Dauvilliers, Y., Krystal, A. D., & Leger, D. (2012). Prevalence and comorbidity of nocturnal wandering in the US adult general population. *Neurology, 78,* 1583–1589. http://doi.org/10.1212/WNL.0b013e3182563be5

Ohayon, M. M., Morselli, P. L., & Guilleminault, C. (1997). Prevalence of nightmares and their relationship to psychopathology and daytime functioning in insomnia subjects. *Sleep, 20,* 340–348. http://doi.org/10.1093/sleep/20.5.340

Ohayon, M. M., & Reynolds, C. F. (2009). Epidemiological and clinical relevance of insomnia diagnosis algorithms according to the DSM-IV and the International Classification of Sleep Disorders (ICSD). *Sleep Medicine, 10,* 952–960. http://doi.org/10.1016/j.sleep.2009.07.008

Okajima, I., Komada, Y., & Inoue, Y. (2011). A meta-analysis on the treatment effectiveness of cognitive behavioral therapy for primary insomnia. *Sleep and Biological Rhythms, 9,* 24–34. http://doi.org/10.1111/j.1479-8425.2010.00481.x

Onen, S. H., Onen, F., Bailly, D., & Parquet, P. (1994). Prevention and treatment of sleep disorders through regulation of sleeping habits. *Presse Medicale, 23,* 485–489.

Ong, J. C., & Crawford, M. R. (2013). Insomnia and obstructive sleep apnea. *Sleep Medicine Clinics, 8,* 389–398. http://doi.org/10.1016/j.jsmc.2013.04.004

Ong, J. C., Manber, R., Segal, Z., Xia, Y., Shapiro, S., & Wyatt, J. K. (2014). A randomized controlled trial of mindfulness meditation for chronic insomnia. *Sleep, 37,* 1553–1563. http://doi.org/10.5665/sleep.4010

Ong, J., & Sholtes, D. (2010). A mindfulness-based approach to the treatment of insomnia. *Journal of Clinical Psychology, 66,* 1175–1184. http://doi.org/10.1002/jclp.20736

Ong, J. C., Ulmer, C. S., & Manber, R. (2012). Improving sleep with mindfulness and acceptance: A metacognitive model of insomnia. *Behaviour Research and Therapy, 50,* 651–660. http://doi.org/10.1016/j.brat.2012.08.001

Papadimitriou, G. N., & Linkowski, P. (2005). Sleep disturbance in anxiety disorders. *International Review of Psychiatry, 17*(4), 229–236. http://doi.org/10.1080/09540260500104524

Parsaik, A. K., Mascarenhas, S. S., Khosh-Chashm, D., Hashmi, A., John, V., Okusaga, O., & Singh, B. (2016). Mortality associated with anxiolytic and hypnotic drugs: A systematic review and meta-analysis. *Australian & New Zealand Journal of Psychiatry, 50,* 520–533.

Perlis, M. L., Giles, D. E., Buysse, D. J., Tu, X., & Kupfer, D. J. (1997). Self-reported sleep disturbance as a prodromal symptom in recurrent depression. *Journal of Affective Disorders, 42,* 209–212. http://doi.org/10.1016/S0165-0327(96)01411-5

Perlis, M. L., Giles, D. E., Mendelson, W. B., Bootzin, R. R., & Wyatt, J. K. (1997). Psychophysiological insomnia: The behavioural model and a neurocognitive perspective. *Journal of Sleep Research, 6,* 179–188. http://doi.org/10.1046/j.1365-2869.1997.00045.x

Perlis, M. L., Merica, H., Smith, M. T., & Giles, D. E. (2001). Beta EEG activity and insomnia. *Sleep Medicine Reviews, 5,* 365–376. http://doi.org/10.1053/smrv.2001.0151

Petrov, M. E. R., Lichstein, K. L., Huisingh, C. E., & Bradley, L. A. (2014). Predictors of adherence to a brief behavioral insomnia intervention: Daily process analysis. *Behavior Therapy, 45,* 430–442. http://doi.org/10.1016/j.beth.2014.01.005

Qaseem, A., Kansagara, D., Forciea, M. A., Cooke, M., & Denberg, T. D. (2016). Management of chronic insomnia disorder in adults: A clinical practice guideline from the American College of Physicians. *Annals of Internal Medicine, 165,* 125–133. http://doi.org/10.7326/M15-2175

Radloff, L. S. (1977). The CES-D scale: A self-report depression scale for research in the general population. *Applied Psychological Measurement, 1,* 385–401. http://doi.org/10.1177/014662167700100306

Reynolds, S. A., & Ebben, M. R. (2017). The cost of insomnia and the benefit of increased access to evidence-based treatment: Cognitive behavioral therapy for insomnia. *Sleep Medicine Clinics, 12,* 39–46. http://doi.org/10.1016/j.jsmc.2016.10.011

Riedel, B. W., & Lichstein, K. L. (2001). Strategies for evaluating adherence to sleep restriction treatment for insomnia. *Behaviour Research and Therapy, 39,* 201–212. http://doi.org/10.1016/S0005-7967(00)00002-4

Riedel, B. W., Lichstein, K. L., & Dwyer, W. O. (1995). Sleep compression and sleep education for older insomniacs: Self-help versus therapist guidance. *Psychology and Aging, 10,* 54–63. http://doi.org/10.1037/0882-7974.10.1.54

Riemann, D., Spiegelhalder, K., Feige, B., Voderholzer, U., Berger, M., Perlis, M., & Nissen, C. (2010). The hyperarousal model of insomnia: A review of the concept and its evidence. *Sleep Medicine Reviews, 14,* 19–31. http://doi.org/10.1016/j.smrv.2009.04.002

Ritterband, L. M., Thorndike, F. P., Ingersoll, K. S., Lord, H. R., Gonder-Frederick, L., Frederick, C., … Morin, C. M. (2017). Effect of a web-based cognitive behavior therapy for insomnia intervention with 1-year follow-up: A randomized clinical trial. *JAMA Psychiatry, 74,* 68–75.

Roehrs, T., & Roth, T. (2001). Sleep, sleepiness, sleep disorders and alcohol use and abuse. *Sleep Medicine Reviews, 5,* 287–297. http://doi.org/10.1053/smrv.2001.0162

Roth, T., Coulouvrat, C., Hajak, G., Lakoma, M. D., Sampson, N. A., Shahly, V., … Kessler, R. C. (2011). Prevalence and perceived health associated with insomnia based on DSM-IV-TR; International statistical classification of diseases and related health problems, tenth revision; and research diagnostic criteria/international classification of sleep disorders, criteria: Results from the America Insomnia Survey. *Biological Psychiatry, 69,* 592–600.

Saletu-Zyhlarz, G., Saletu, B., Anderer, P., Brandstätter, N., Frey, R., Gruber, G., … Linzmayer, L. (1997). Nonorganic insomnia in generalized anxiety disorder. *Neuropsychobiology, 36,* 117–129. http://doi.org/10.1159/000119373

Sateia, M. J., Doghramji, K., Hauri, P. J., & Morin, C. M. (2000). Evaluation of chronic insomnia: An American Academy of Sleep Medicine review. *Sleep, 23,* 243–308. http://doi.org/10.1093/sleep/23.2.11

Savard, J., & Morin, C. M. (2001). Insomnia in the context of cancer: A review of a neglected problem. *Journal of Clinical Oncology, 19,* 895–908. http://doi.org/10.1200/JCO.2001.19.3.895

Savard, J., & Savard, M. H. (2013). Insomnia and cancer: prevalence, nature, and nonpharmacologic treatment. *Sleep Medicine Clinics, 8,* 373–387. http://doi.org/10.1016/j.jsmc.2013.04.006

Schutte-Rodin, S., Broch, L., Buysse, D., Dorsey, C., & Sateia, M. (2008). Clinical guideline for the evaluation and management of chronic insomnia in adults. *Journal of Clinical Sleep Medicine, 4,* 487–504.

Shahly, V., Berglund, P. A., Coulouvrat, C., Fitzgerald, T., Hajak, G., Roth, T., … Kessler, R. C. (2012). The associations of insomnia with costly workplace accidents and errors: Results from the America Insomnia Survey. *Archives of General Psychiatry, 69,* 1054–1063. http://doi.org/10.1001/archgenpsychiatry.2011.2188

Shear, K., Belnap, B. H., Mazumdar, S., Houck, P., & Rollman, B. L. (2006). Generalized anxiety disorder severity scale (GADSS): A preliminary validation study. *Depression and Anxiety, 23,* 77–82. http://doi.org/10.1002/da.20149

Silver, R., & LeSauter, J. (2008). Circadian and homeostatic factors in arousal. *Annals of the New York Academy of Sciences, 1129,* 263–274. http://doi.org/10.1196/annals.1417.032

Smith, M. T., Huang, M. I., & Manber, R. (2005). Cognitive behavior therapy for chronic insomnia occurring within the context of medical and psychiatric disorders. *Clinical Psychology Review, 25,* 559–592. http://doi.org/10.1016/j.cpr.2005.04.004

Smith, M. T., Perlis, M. L., Park, A., Smith, M. S., Pennington, J., Giles, D. E., & Buysse, D. J. (2002). Comparative meta-analysis of pharmacotherapy and behavior therapy for persistent insomnia. *American Journal of Psychiatry, 159,* 5–11. http://doi.org/10.1176/appi.ajp.159.1.5

Sobell, L. C., & Sobell, M. B. (2003). Using motivational interviewing techniques to talk with clients about their alcohol use. *Cognitive and Behavioral Practice, 10,* 214–221. http://doi.org/10.1016/S1077-7229(03)80033-0

Soehner, A. M., Kaplan, K. A., & Harvey, A. G. (2013). Insomnia comorbid to severe psychiatric illness. *Sleep Medicine Clinics, 8,* 361–371. http://doi.org/10.1016/j.jsmc.2013.04.007

Spielberger, C. D., Gorsuch, R. L., Lushene, R., Vagg, P. R., & Jacobs, G. A. (1983). *Manual for the State-Trait Anxiety Inventory.* Palo Alto, CA: Consulting Psychologists Press.

Spielman, A. J. (1986). Assessment of insomnia. *Clinical Psychology Review, 6,* 11–25. http://doi.org/10.1016/0272-7358(86)90015-2

Spielman, A. J., Saskin, P., & Thorpy, M. J. (1987). Treatment of chronic insomnia by restriction of time in bed. *Sleep, 10,* 45–56.

Spielman, A. J., Yang, C., & Glovinsky, P. B. (2011). Assessment techniques for insomnia. In M. H. Kryger, T. Roth, & W. C. Dement (Eds.), *Principles and practice of sleep medicine* (pp. 1632–1645). St. Louis, MO: Elsevier Books.

Spitzer, R. L., Kroenke, K., Williams, J. B., & Löwe, B. (2006). A brief measure for assessing generalized anxiety disorder: The GAD-7. *Archives of Internal Medicine, 166,* 1092–1097. http://doi.org/10.1001/archinte.166.10.1092

Stepanski, E. J., & Wyatt, J. K. (2003). Use of sleep hygiene in the treatment of insomnia. *Sleep Medicine Reviews, 7,* 215–225. http://doi.org/10.1053/smrv.2001.0246

Swift, N., Stewart, R., Andiappan, M., Smith, A., Espie, C. A., & Brown, J. S. (2012). The effectiveness of community day-long CBT-I workshops for participants with insomnia symptoms: A randomised controlled trial. *Journal of Sleep Research, 21,* 270–280. http://doi.org/10.1111/j.1365-2869.2011.00940.x

Tannenbaum, C., Diaby, V., Singh, D., Perreault, S., Luc, M., & Vasiliadis, H. M. (2015). Sedative-hypnotic medicines and falls in community-dwelling older adults: A cost-effectiveness (decision-tree) analysis from a US Medicare perspective. *Drugs & Aging, 32,* 305–314.

Taylor, D. J., Lichstein, K. L., Durrence, H. H., Reidel, B. W., & Bush, A. J. (2005). Epidemiology of insomnia, depression, and anxiety. *Sleep, 28,* 1457–1464. http://doi.org/10.1093/sleep/28.11.1457

Taylor, D. J., Mallory, L. J., Lichstein, K. L., Durrence, H., Riedel, B. W., & Bush, A. J. (2007). Comorbidity of chronic insomnia with medical problems. *Sleep, 30,* 213–218. http://doi.org/10.1093/sleep/30.2.213

Taylor, D. J., & Pruiksma, K. E. (2014). Cognitive and behavioural therapy for insomnia (CBT-I) in psychiatric populations: A systematic review. *International Review of Psychiatry, 26,* 205–213. http://doi.org/10.3109/09540261.2014.902808

Taylor, H. L., Hailes, H. P., & Ong, J. (2015). Third-wave therapies for insomnia. *Current Sleep Medicine Reports, 1,* 166–176. http://doi.org/10.1007/s40675-015-0020-1

Trauer, J. M., Qian, M. Y., Doyle, J. S., Rajaratnam, S. M., & Cunnington, D. (2015). Cognitive behavioral therapy for chronic insomnia: A systematic review and meta-analysis. *Annals of Internal Medicine, 163,* 191–204. http://doi.org/10.7326/M14-2841

Tremblay, V., Savard, J., & Ivers, H. (2009). Predictors of the effect of cognitive behavioral therapy for chronic insomnia comorbid with breast cancer. *Journal of Consulting and Clinical Psychology, 77,* 742–750. http://doi.org/10.1037/a0015492

Van Straten, A., & Cuijpers, P. (2009). Self-help therapy for insomnia: A meta-analysis. *Sleep Medicine Reviews, 13,* 61–71. http://doi.org/10.1016/j.smrv.2008.04.006

Vincent, N. K., & Hameed, H. (2003). Relation between adherence and outcome in the group treatment of insomnia. *Behavioral Sleep Medicine, 1,* 125–139. http://doi.org/10.1207/S15402010BSM0103_1

Vincent, N., Lewycky, S., & Finnegan, H. (2008). Barriers to engagement in sleep restriction and stimulus control in chronic insomnia. *Journal of Consulting and Clinical Psychology, 76,* 820–828. http://doi.org/10.1037/0022-006X.76.5.820

Vincent, N., & Walsh, K. (2013). Stepped care for insomnia: An evaluation of implementation in routine practice. *Journal of Clinical Sleep Medicine, 9,* 227–234. http://doi.org/10.5664/jcsm.2484

Wade, A. G. (2011). The societal costs of insomnia. *Neuropsychiatric Disease and Treatment, 7,* 1–18.

Walsh, J. K., Coulouvrat, C., Hajak, G., Lakoma, M. D., Petukhova, M., Roth, T., … Kessler, R. C. (2011). Nighttime insomnia symptoms and perceived health in the America Insomnia Survey (AIS). *Sleep, 34,* 997–1011. http://doi.org/10.5665/SLEEP.1150

Wohlgemuth, W. K., Edinger, J. D., Fins, A. I., & Sullivan, R. J. (1999). How many nights are enough? The short-term stability of sleep parameters in elderly insomniacs and normal sleepers. *Psychophysiology, 36,* 233–244. http://doi.org/10.1111/1469-8986.3620233

Wong, M. Y., Ree, M. J., & Lee, C. W. (2015). Enhancing CBT for chronic insomnia: A randomised clinical trial of additive components of mindfulness or cognitive therapy. *Clinical Psychology & Psychotherapy, 23,* 377–385. http://doi.org/10.1002/cpp.1980

World Health Organization. (2018). *International classification of diseases for mortality and morbidity statistics* (11th ed., stable version for implementation). Geneva, Switzerland: Author. Retrieved from https://icd.who.int/browse11/l-m/en

Wyatt, J. K. (2004). Delayed sleep phase syndrome: Pathophysiology and treatment options. *Sleep, 27,* 1195–1203. http://doi.org/10.1093/sleep/27.6.1195

Zachariae, R., Lyby, M. S., Ritterband, L. M., & O'Toole, M. S. (2016). Efficacy of internet-delivered cognitive-behavioral therapy for insomnia – a systematic review and meta-analysis of randomized controlled trials. *Sleep Medicine Reviews, 30,* 1–10. http://doi.org/10.1016/j.smrv.2015.10.004

Zayfert, C., & DeViva, J. C. (2004). Residual insomnia following cognitive behavioral therapy for PTSD. *Journal of Traumatic Stress, 17,* 69–73. http://doi.org/10.1023/B:JOTS.0000014679.31799.e7

Zhang, J. X., Liu, X. H., Xie, X. H., Zhao, D., Shan, M. S., Zhang, X. L., … Cui, H. (2015). Mindfulness-based stress reduction for chronic insomnia in adults older than 75 years: A randomized, controlled, single-blind clinical trial. *EXPLORE: The Journal of Science and Healing, 11,* 180–185.

Zung, W. W. (1965). A self-rating depression scale. *Archives of General Psychiatry, 12,* 63–70. http://doi.org/10.1001/archpsyc.1965.01720310065008

8

Appendix: Tools and Resources

Appendix 1: Recommended Resource Websites
Appendix 2: Insomnia Assessment
Appendix 3: Sleep Diary and Instructions
Appendix 4: Sample Sleep Diary of Patient L.F. and Calculation Instructions
Appendix 5: Clinician Psychoeducation Sample Script
Appendix 6: Guidelines for Better Sleep

Recommended Resource Websites

Sleep Education

http://www.sleepeducation.org/
The American Academy of Sleep Medicine (AASM) is the largest organization of sleep specialists in the US and the accrediting body for sleep centers. The AASM has developed a website designed to provide the public and clinicians with information about many types of sleep disorders. It also provides a search engine to locate AASM-accredited sleep centers.

Society of Behavioral Sleep Medicine

https://www.behavioralsleep.org/
According to its website, the Society of Behavioral Sleep Medicine is "an interdisciplinary organization committed to advancing the scientific approach to studying the behavioral, psychological, and physiological dimensions of sleep and sleep disorders and the application of this knowledge to the betterment of individuals and societies worldwide." It provides information about adult and childhood sleep disorders, with an emphasis on behavioral interventions for these disorders. The site also includes information about educational opportunities and training resources for clinicians.

Insomnia Assessment

The purpose of the assessment presented on the following pages is to specifically evaluate the patient's sleep complaint. In addition, there are items to screen for a variety of sleep disorders that may present with insomnia complaints. The reader is referred to Chapter 3 for more detailed descriptions of these differential diagnoses. Clinicians should also incorporate a standard evaluation of the patient's medical, psychiatric, social and family history. Assessment of these additional aspects of the patient's history is not included in the following questionnaire.

Insomnia History

1. Describe your current sleep problem:

____

____

____

How long have you had this problem? ______________________________

How long have you been concerned with this sleep problem? ______________________

Has the severity of the sleep problem changed over time? ☐ No ☐ Yes

If yes, **describe** ______________________________________

____

____

When you were a child, did you experience any sleep difficulties? ☐ No ☐ Yes

If yes, **describe** ______________________________________

____

____

2. What do you think contributes to your sleep problem? Can you identify the cause of your sleep difficulties?

____

____

____

3. How many hours of sleep do you feel you need each night to feel rested? ______________

Generally, how many hours of sleep do you get a night? ______________________

Think about nights when you consider you slept well, how many hours would you say you sleep on those good nights? ______________________________

What about on bad nights, how many hours would you say you sleep on those nights? ______________

4. What would you estimate is the length of time you generally take to fall asleep? ____________________

How long might that be on a good night? ____________________

How long might that be on a bad night? ____________________

5. Consider your awakenings throughout the night. After falling asleep, how many awakenings would you estimate you experience on a bad night? ____________________

What about on a good night? ____________________

How long would you say each of your awakenings last? ____________________

6. How many times per week do you have difficulty:

Falling asleep ____________________ (times/week)

Returning to sleep ____________________ (times/week)

Waking up too early ____________________ (times/week)

7. How do you generally feel during the day (e.g., concentration or memory difficulties, fatigue or irritability)?

____

____

Is it different depending on whether you've had a good night or a bad night of sleep?

Describe: ____________________

____

____

Sleep Habits

8. What time do you normally get into bed? ____________________

What time do you normally try to go to sleep? ____________________

What time do you normally wake up? ____________________

What time do you get out of bed? ______________________________

Are these times regular/consistent each day? ☐ No ☐ Yes

Describe: ______________________________

____

____

Would you prefer your bedtime and/or waketime at later or earlier times than those listed above?

☐ No ☐ Yes

If yes, when would you prefer? ______________________________

____

9. Do you take naps? ☐ No ☐ Yes

How many times each week? ______________________________

How long do your naps last? ______________________________

10. Indicate how frequently you engage in the activities listed below *while you are in bed or in your bedroom:*

1 = Not at all (0 times per week)
2 = Some of the time (1–3 times per week)
3 = Most of the time (4–6 times per week)
4 = All of the time (7 times per week)

a. Watch television ________

b. Use electronic devices ________

c. Read ________

d. Eat ________

e. Work or study ________

f. Talk on the phone ________

11. On a scale from 1 to 10, what number best reflects how much difficulty you have relaxing your body at bedtime.

No difficulty				Some difficulty					Great difficulty
1	2	3	4	5	6	7	8	9	10

12. On a scale from 1 to 10, what number best reflects how much difficulty you have "slowing down" or "turning off your mind" while trying to sleep.

No difficulty				Some difficulty					Great difficulty
1	2	3	4	5	6	7	8	9	10

External Factors Which Influence Sleep

13. Do you have a bedpartner? ☐ No ☐ Yes

If yes, does having a bedpartner interfere with your sleep (e.g., snoring, movement, etc.)?

Describe: ______________________________

____

____

14. Do you find the temperature, noise level, or lighting in your sleep environment bothersome?

☐ No ☐ Yes

If yes, **describe:** ______________________________

____

15. Indicate how frequently and at what time(s) of the day you consume the following during the week:

1 = Not at all (0 times per week)
2 = Some of the time (1–3 times per week)
3 = Most of the time (4–6 times per week)
4 = All of the time (7 times per week)

	Frequency	Time(s) of Day
a. Coffee (with caffeine)	__________	__________
b. Tea (with caffeine)	__________	__________
c. Soft drinks (with caffeine)	__________	__________
d. Energy drinks	__________	__________
e. Alcohol	__________	__________
f. Cigarettes or tobacco products	__________	__________
g. Other drugs	__________	__________

Symptoms of Comorbid Sleep Disorders

16. On the scale below, rate how sleepy you have been feeling during the day (e.g., fighting sleep, struggling to stay awake):

Alert — Somewhat sleepy — Cannot stay awake

1	2	3	4	5	6	7	8	9	10

Does the sleepiness depend on whether you've had a good night or a bad night of sleep? ☐ No ☐ Yes

Describe: ____

____

____

17. How many times during a typical week do you have a problem with severe sleepiness (feeling very sleepy or struggling to stay awake during the daytime)? ____________________

18. Do you snore? ☐ No ☐ Yes

Do others complain about your snoring? ☐ No ☐ Yes

19. Has anyone ever told you that you seem to stop breathing or to gasp for breath during your sleep?

☐ No ☐ Yes If yes, how often has this been noted? ____________________

____

20. How many times per month, on average (if none, write "0")

Has someone noticed your legs twitching during your sleep? ______ times per month

At bedtime, do you experience a strong urge to move your legs? ______times per month

Does this sensation in your legs make it hard for you to fall asleep? ☐ No ☐ Yes

Do you sleepwalk? ______times per month

Do you have nightmares? ______times per month

21. What times of the day or night do you work? ______________________________

____

22. Do your work hours change or rotate? ☐ No ☐ Yes

Describe: ____

____

____

23. How often do you travel across time zones (number of times per month)?

____

Attempts to Reduce Insomnia Symptoms

24. Currently, how many times during the month do you use medication to help you fall asleep? __________

What medication(s) do you use? ______________________________________

____

25. How many times during the month do you drink alcohol to help you fall asleep? ______________

On those nights when you do drink alcohol to help you sleep, how much do you drink? ______________

____

26. What treatments have you tried in the past to help you sleep?

____

____

How well did those treatments work?

____

____

27. Is there anything else that you have tried to help you sleep better?

____

____

Motivation and Readiness for Treatment

Please answer the next two questions with regard to the importance and confidence you have in changing your sleep difficulties.

28. At this moment, how important is your goal to achieve better sleep at night?

0	25	50	75	100
Not important at all	Less important than most of the other things I would like to achieve now	About as important as most of the other things I would like to achieve now	More important than most of the other things I would like to achieve now	Most important thing in my life I would like to achieve now

The importance of my goal is ____________________________

Now ask yourself the following question:

What competing priorities, if any, could interfere with you achieving your goal?

____

____

____

____

____

29. At this moment, how confident are you that you can change your sleep difficulties?

0------------------------25------------------------50------------------------75------------------------100

Not important at all	Less important than most of the other things I would like to achieve now	About as important as most of the other things I would like to achieve now	More important than most of the other things I would like to achieve now	Most important thing in my life I would like to achieve now

I am ______% confident that I will achieve my goal.

Now ask yourself the following question:

What obstacles, if any, might you encounter that could interfere with you achieving your goal?

____

____

____

____

30. What prompted you to seek treatment at this time?

____

____

____

____

31. On a scale from 1 to 10, what number best reflects how ready you were *6 months ago* and how ready you are *now* to change the behaviors that prompted you to seek treatment?

Definitely not ready to change | Somewhat ready to change | Definitely ready to change

1	2	3	4	5	6	7	8	9	10

31a. ______ 6 months ago **31b. ______Today**

Sleep Diary of ____________________

	SAMPLE							
Day of the Week (When You Woke Up)	Monday							
Calendar Date	*3/18/13*							
1. Yesterday I napped from ___ to___ (note time of all naps).	*1:30–2:45 PM*							
2. Last night I took ___ mg. of ___ , or ___ of alcohol as a sleep aid.	*Ambien 5 mg*							
3. Last night I got into bed at ___ (AM or PM?)	*11:00 PM*							
4. Last night I turned off the lights and attempted to fall asleep at ___ (AM or PM?)	*11:30 PM*							
5. After turning off the lights, it took me about ___ minutes to fall sleep.	*40 min*							
6. I woke from sleep ___ times. (Do not count your final awakening here)	*2 times*							
7. In total, how long did these awakenings last?	*70 min*							
8. Today I woke up at ___ (AM or PM?) NOTE this is your **final** awakening.	*6:30 AM*							
9. Today I got out of bed for the day at ___ (AM or PM?).	*7:15 AM*							
10. The quality of last night's sleep was: 1 = very poor 4 = good 2 = poor 5 = excellent 3 = fair	*3*							
11. When I awoke today I felt: 1 = not all rested 4 = rested 2 = slightly rested 5 = well-rested 3 = somewhat rested	*2*							
Time in bed								
Total sleep time								
Sleep efficiency (%)								

Instructions for Completing the Sleep Diary

You should complete the Sleep Diary shortly after awakening each morning.

CAUTION!

Do **NOT** worry about whether you are being totally accurate. Sometimes, people will try to keep track of their sleep during the night (for example, watching the clock or keeping a record of each time they wake up.) DO NOT DO THIS. Such an approach interferes with your normal sleep pattern. Instead, forget about the Diary during the night. When you wake up in the morning, complete the Diary by giving us your best estimate on each question.

EACH MORNING, take the Sleep Diary and complete it according to the following instructions.

Fill in your NAME, YESTERDAY'S DATE, and YESTERDAY'S DAY OF THE WEEK on the top of the Sleep Diary in the appropriate box.

1. If you took a nap yesterday, estimate how long you slept during your nap. If you took several naps, add your times together and fill in the total number of minutes you slept. If you did not take a nap, write N/A (not applicable).
2. Write the name and dosage of any medication or the amount of alcohol you took to help you sleep.
3. Write the time that you got into bed. This may not be the time you began "trying" to fall asleep.
4. Give the time you turned off the lights and tried to sleep last night.
5. Estimate the amount of time it took you to fall asleep.
6. Estimate the number of times you woke up during the night. DO NOT count your final awakening in the morning.
7. If you awoke during the night, estimate the total time you were awake. If you awoke more than once, add up the total time that you were awake.
8. Estimate when you woke up for the final time.
9. Estimate the time you actually were out of bed.

10–11. Give your rating for each of these questions.

Sample Sleep Diary of Patient L.F. (Case Vignette in Chapter 5)

Day of the Week (When You Woke Up)	Monday	Friday	Saturday	Sunday	Monday	Tuesday	Wednesday	Thursday
Calendar Date	*3/18/13*	12/2/16	12/3/16	12/4/16	12/5/16	12/6/16	12/7/16	12/8/16
1. Yesterday I napped from ___ to___ (note time of all naps).	*1:30–2:45 PM*	N/A	N/A	N/A	N/A	N/A	N/A	N/A
2. Last night I took ___ mg. of ___ , or ___ of alcohol as a sleep aid.	*Ambien 5 mg*	N/A	N/A	N/A	N/A	N/A	N/A	N/A
3. Last night I got into bed at ___ (AM or PM?)	*11:00 PM*	10:00 PM	12:00 AM	12:00 AM	1:00 AM	10:00 PM	9:30 PM	11:00 PM
4. Last night I turned off the lights and attempted to fall asleep at ___ (AM or PM?)	*11:30 PM*	10:30 PM	12:00 AM	12:00 AM	1:00 AM	10:00 PM	10:00 PM	11:30 PM
5. After turning off the lights, it took me about ___ minutes to fall sleep.	*40 min*	60 min	20 min	15 min	20 min	60 min	60 min	30 min
6. I woke from sleep ___ times. (Do not count your final awakening here)	*2 times*	2 times	3 times	4 times	1 times	5 times	4 times	1 Times
7. In total, how long did these awakenings last?	*70 min*	30 min	60 min	90 min	15 min	90 min	60 min	30 min
8. Today I woke up at ___ (AM or PM?) NOTE this is your **final** awakening.	*6:30 AM*	6:00 AM	6:30 AM	6:00 AM	8:45 AM	6:30 AM	6:30 AM	6:30 AM
9. Today I got out of bed for the day at ___ (AM or PM?).	*7:15 AM*	6:00 AM	6:30 AM	6:30 AM	9:00 AM	8:00 AM	7:00 AM	7:30 AM
10. The quality of last night's sleep was: 1 = very poor 4 = good 2 = poor 5 = excellent 3 = fair	*3*	2	2	2	3	1	1	2
11. When I awoke today I felt: 1 = not all rested 4 = rested 2 = slightly rested 5 = well-rested 3 = somewhat rested	*2*	2	1	1	2	1	1	2
Time in bed		450	390	390	480	600	540	480
Total sleep time		360	310	255	430	360	390	360
Sleep efficiency (%)		80%	79%	65%	90%	60%	72%	75%

Sleep Diary Calculation Instructions

Item numbers referred to in these calculations correspond to the completed Sleep Diary of Patient L.F. on the previous page.

1. **Total time in bed (TIB) → calculate for** each day

   Total TIB is calculated by finding the number of minutes between the time the patient attempts to fall asleep in bed (Item 4) and the time the patient gets out of bed (Item 9).

   Example for the date Friday 12/2/2016:
   Item 4 = 10:30 p.m.
   Item 9 = 6:00 a.m.
   7 hrs 30 min → 420 min + 30 min = 450 min → TIB = 450 min

2. **Total sleep time (TST) → calculate for each day**

   TST is calculated by subtracting the total time a patient is awake during the night from the TIB, as follows

   a. Step 1 → Total time it takes to fall asleep (Item 5, total minutes) + Total for all awakenings during the night (Item 7, total minutes) + Total for difference between time of final awakening and time out of bed (Item 9 – Item 8, total minutes).
   b. Step 2 → Subtract the amount from Step 1 from the TIB calculated above.

   Example:
   Item 5 = 60 min to fall asleep
   Item 7 = 30 min of awakenings
   Item 9 – Item 8 = 0 min (awoke at 6:00 a.m. and got out of bed at 6:00 a.m.)
   Step 1 → Item 5 + Item 7 + Diff. b/w Item 9 and 8 = 60 + 30 + 0 = 90
   Step 2 → TIB – Step 1 total= 450 – 90 = 360

3. **Sleep efficiency percentage (SE%) → calculate for each day**

   a. TST/TIB = SE (360/450 = .80) → example of a daily SE
   b. Calculate *average SE* = SE for each day totaled / number of days
   c. Average SE = average TST / average TIB
   d. Multiply this average SE by 100 to get the average SE%

4. **TIB prescription**

   a. Calculate average TST (TST for each day totaled / number of days).
      Average TST = (360 + 310 + 255 + 430 + 360 + 390 + 360) / 7 = 352
   b. Calculate recommended TIB by adding 30 min to average TST (352 + 30 = 382 min or approximately 6 hrs and 22 min).
   c. Ask patient to choose a standard wake-up time to use *every day.*
   d. Set bedtime recommendation by subtracting the amount of time of TIB prescription (382 min) from the selected standard wake-up time. Remember that the bedtime is only a recommended time. That is, the patient should *never go to bed before this time* but should only go to bed at this time *if* they are already sleepy, otherwise they should wait to go to sleep later when feeling sleepy.
   e. Have patient take active role in setting standard waketime and bedtime in order to arrive at a desirable schedule.

5. **TIB adjustments during treatment**

   a. If average SE% ≥ 85% for previous week AND patient reports feeling too sleepy during the day, *then add* 15 min to initial TIB prescription for the next week.
   b. If average SE% < 80% for previous week *then subtract* 15 min from initial TIB prescription for the next week.

Clinician Psychoeducation Sample Script

The following script provides the clinician with sample language that can be used to explain the psychoeducation concepts. It is important that this information be conveyed in a manner that the patient understands, as it builds the foundation for the instructions that will be laid out for the patient to follow.

The treatment you are undertaking to help reduce your sleep difficulties is called *cognitive behavioral therapy for insomnia*, or CBT-I. Over the next few weeks of treatment, you will be modifying various behaviors that affect your sleep, and some of the things we will be discussing now will help you understand why you are making these changes.

How Does Age Affect Sleep?

Our bodies undergo many changes as we grow older. These changes can affect the ways they work. Sleep is one of these processes that change with age. As we age, we may find ourselves experiencing more awakenings throughout the night. Also, as we age, the amount of time that we spend in the deeper stages of sleep is reduced. In addition, we may find ourselves getting sleepy earlier in the evening and waking up earlier than we used to. These changes may cause us to feel less refreshed when we wake up in the mornings. It's important to keep these things in mind as you consider your sleep. What are your expectations now for a good night's sleep? Are you hoping to sleep the way you did when you were much younger? Are your goals for treatment consistent with these natural sleep changes?

How Much Sleep Do You Really Need?

How much sleep do you need? Most people will answer this question by saying they need 8 hrs of sleep. In fact, most adults up to 64 years of age need between 7 and 9 hrs, while most adults over the age of 64 require 7 to 8 hrs of sleep. Nevertheless, these numbers only serve as a guide. Indeed, there is no easy answer to how much sleep any one person needs. The way we answer this question is by asking, "How much sleep do you need to feel rested and refreshed when you wake up?" Sometimes, this is not a satisfactory answer for most folks because figuring out the answer takes time and effort. However, as you follow the treatment recommendations and begin adapting your sleep schedule and making behavior changes, you will find that gradually your sleep will improve, and through our work together, you will be able to get a much better sense of what your unique sleep needs are.

How Does Your Body Play a Role in Assisting You to Fall and Stay Asleep?

Two systems in your body are very important in influencing your sleeping and waking times. The first is our sleep drive. Simply put, our bodies are wired to sleep when we have been awake for a long period of time. Throughout our waking hours, our brain is naturally building up this drive to sleep. The longer we stay awake, the greater the intensity of that drive, so that eventually our need for sleep overwhelms the body's ability to remain awake. After enough hours of being awake, we have no choice but to sleep. The second function is associated with our body's clock, which keeps us on a daily rhythm. This internal clock helps to keep our brain alert and awake during daytime hours and quiets down during the night so that sleep comes easier. These two systems work together to help keep us on a regular 24-hr rhythm of being awake and alert during the day and sleeping at night. How often do you alter the times you get up in the morning and go to bed at night? How frequently do you nap during the day? These behaviors can interfere with the normal functioning of these systems and make it much more difficult for us to sleep well.

Why Is Spending Too Much Time in Bed Perhaps Not a Good Strategy for You?

It is not unusual for someone with insomnia to stay in bed later after a poor night's sleep or decide to go to bed earlier than normal after a couple of nights of disrupted sleep. Many times those who experience severe symptoms of insomnia will routinely spend longer periods of time in bed in the hopes of getting enough sleep each night. Unfortunately, this strategy is ineffective, and staying in bed for long periods of time can be seriously counterproductive. Our brains are fantastic learning machines. In this particular instance, however, they learn to connect the bed with being awake. If we consistently spend too much time in bed – more than what is necessary to meet our individual sleep need – our sleep will begin to spread out over this extended period in bed. This means that in between sleep periods, we find ourselves spending more time awake. Not only are these awakenings inconvenient, but they can also be extremely frustrating and anxiety provoking to some. Indeed, the increased arousal experienced around these awakenings can train us to relate the bed with being awake. Although this process is unintentional and happens automatically, it can further aggravate the amount of time we spend awake in bed. So while spending more time in bed may seem like a helpful solution to insomnia, it will most likely make the problem worse.

Why is the Bed Only for Sleeping?

Engaging in waking activities in bed (and even in the bedroom) can unintentionally train us that it's ok to be awake in bed. Reading, watching television, playing on a smartphone, or talking on the phone are a few examples of the many waking activities that individuals often do in bed. Usually we are hoping to get drowsy while doing these activities in bed, but these things require alertness. For someone experiencing insomnia, it is best to retrain ourselves to associate the bed with only sleepiness and sleeping. This means all other activities requiring alertness (with the exception of sex or being sick) should be left outside of the bed and bedroom. This way, over time, the bed and bedroom will be connected with sleep, and bothersome awakenings will diminish.

Guidelines for Better Sleep

The following handout can be provided to the patient after the psychoeducation component is completed. It can function as a platform for discussing the various guidelines that they will follow during treatment. Additionally, the points included in the handout serve to reinforce the information covered during the psychoeducation module. By providing the handout, the patient can refer back to these items throughout the week and recall the reasons they are being asked to follow the guidelines. The individual items along with their rationale should be reviewed with the patient.

Guidelines for Better Sleep

For sounder, more reliable sleep, follow all of the guidelines below.

1. **Establish a standard wake-up time AND stick to it every day no matter what your sleep is like on any particular night.**
   a. You cannot force yourself to go to sleep, BUT you can control the time when you wake up.
   b. The goal is to try to avoid different wake-up times and to establish a standard sleep–wake schedule because constantly changing your sleep–wake schedule can disrupt your sleep.
   c. By waking up at the same time every day, you'll notice that you begin to get sleepy at about the same time each night, and over the course of time, this will help you to obtain the sleep you need.

2. **Never spend long periods of time awake in bed. When you are unable to sleep, get up and go to another room. Return to your bed only when you feel sleepy again. Continue to do this each time you find yourself spending long periods of time awake in bed.**
   a. Being awake for a long period of time in bed can cause you to feel frustrated, and you may find yourself worrying about your lack of sleep. This inevitably makes it harder for you to fall asleep.
   b. Give yourself *20 minutes* to fall asleep. If you do not fall asleep within 20 minutes, get up, go to another room and only return to the bed once you feel sleepy again.

3. **Avoid naps.**
   a. Naps during the day may reduce your sleepiness and fatigue but also can delay the time when you start to feel sleepy at night.

4. **Use the bed only for sleeping. Do NOT read, watch TV, use electronic devices, eat, etc. Sexual activity or illness are the exceptions to this guideline.**
   a. By doing these activities in bed, you are training yourself (not intentionally) to be awake in bed when you engage in these wakeful activities.
   b. If you consistently avoid these activities, the bed will gradually become linked with sleep, and you will find it easier to fall asleep.
   c. If your bedpartner does wakeful activities in bed ask them to alter these activities during the treatment.

5. **Avoid worrying, thinking, planning, etc. in bed. If such mental activities come on automatically in bed, then get up and go to another room, stay up until you feel sleepy and the mental activities don't disrupt your sleep. Once in bed, get up again if sleep does not come quickly (20 minutes).**
   a. Remember, doing wakeful activities in bed involves unintentionally training yourself to be awake in bed.
   b. Try to schedule time during the day (or in the early evening) to focus on these mental activities with the goal of anticipating, planning ahead, and working through some of the worries. If these worries are reviewed during the day, there is less chance of having them in bed or that they may keep you up at night.

6. **The amount of time you spend in bed should match the amount of sleep you need. In order to do this, go to bed only when you are sleepy but not before the earliest bedtime recommended for you below.**
   a. Research shows that spending too much time in bed leads to broken or fragmented sleep patterns which can worsen the sleep difficulties.
   b. With the aid of a sleep diary, your therapist will help determine the most appropriate time for you to spend in bed each night.
   c. During the treatment you and your therapist will collaborate and decide the amount of time that you will spend in bed along with the wake-up time and bedtime that you will use daily.

Based on the discussion I have had with my therapist, I will use ________________ as my routine wake-up time; I agree to be out of bed by this time each morning. Also, I agree that I will not go to bed before __________________ so that I do not spend too much time in bed each night.

Other Helpful Hints That May Improve Your Sleep

1. **Limit your intake of coffee, tea, soft drinks, chocolate, and other caffeinated substances.**
   a. Caffeine delays sleep onset and may produce broken sleep patterns.
   b. If you do use caffeinated substances, avoid consuming these after 2:00 or 3:00 p.m.

2. **Avoid alcohol use as a sleep aid.**
   a. Alcohol can produce broken sleep patterns.
   b. Avoid drinking alcohol close to bedtime.

3. **Reduce loud noises during the night with earplugs or a sound-screening device (fan, air conditioner).**
   a. External noises can interfere with your ability to fall asleep or stay asleep.

4. **Control the temperatures in your bedroom.**
   a. Temperatures above 75 degrees Fahrenheit may cause broken sleep.
   b. Try to avoid it being too cold or too hot.

5. **Participate in regular aerobic exercise.**
   a. Exercise may help deepen your sleep.
   b. Exercising close to bedtime, however, can make it harder for you to fall asleep. Therefore, exercise no later than late afternoon or early evening.

6. **Avoid going to bed either hungry or too full.**
   a. Your attention will be on your sensation of hunger or the discomfort associated with being too full rather than on sleep.

7. **Minimize exposure to bright light in the hour before bedtime or during the night.**
   a. Light from electronic devices (cell phones, tablets, and computers) interfere with your ability to fall asleep and may make you stay awake longer in the middle of the night.